D0452051

HONEY
The Gourmet
Medicine

HONEY
The Gourmet
Medicine

Joe Traynor

KOVAK BOOKS
P.O. Box 1422, Bakersfield, CA 93302

ORDER FROM:
ATLASBOOKS.COM
800.247.6553

LAKE TAHOE COMMUNITY COLLEGE
LIBRARY AND MEDIA SERVICES

HONEY
The Gourmet
Medicine

Copyright © 2002 by Joe Traynor

All rights reserved. No part of this book may be reproduced, stored in a retrieval system or transmitted in any form by any means, electronic, mechanical, photocopy, recording or otherwise, without the prior permission of the author, except as provided by USA copyright law.

Edited by Mark Goodin

Printed in the United States of America

ISBN: 0-9604704-1-7

For Nema

And dedicated to U.S. honey producers,
who provide the finest tasting
food-medicine on Earth.

■ ACKNOWLEDGMENTS

This book would not have been written had it not been for the groundbreaking reviews by Peter Molan. Like others, I had heard anecdotal claims of the medicinal benefits of honey for years, but Molan's reviews (and his own work) showed that these anecdotes should be taken seriously.

The International Bee Research Association (IBRA) provided a world of information on honey, and the trilogy of books on honey by the association's first director, Eva Crane, form the foundation of any work on the subject. The National Honey Board also provided much useful information.

Thanks to both Peter Molan and the International Bee Research Association for granting permission to include the references Molan cited in his honey-as-medicine reviews.

Mark Goodin, proprietor of Semicolon Editing Service, Mariposa, California, provided invaluable assistance in rewording and reworking a number of passages herein. Virtually all of Mark's tactful suggestions are incorporated in the book. Many thanks, Mark!

Daniel Pouesi of KIN Publications deserves all the credit for making this book a thing of beauty. His willingness to jump right in and completely take care of all the graphic and design work took a lot of worry out of the creation of this book. Thank you, Daniel!

Thanks to everyone at BookMasters for their help and patience for putting this book together.

Two libraries at the University of California, Davis, were indispensable sources of information: the main library and the Health Sciences library. Many solid studies on the medicinal benefits of honey lie—unread—on the shelves of the latter.

Adrian Wenner reviewed the manuscript and provided many useful suggestions. I alone, of course, am responsible for any misstatements herein, however any misstatements that might be subject to legal proceedings are the responsibility of my able assistant, Sammy "The Snake" Simoni.

■

NOTE:

This book is intended only as a guide to the medicinal benefits of honey, not as a medical manual for self-treatment. Seek competent help if you suspect you have a medical problem. The information presented in this book is intended to acquaint you with the potential medicinal benefits of honey; it is not intended to substitute, nor *should* it substitute, for any treatment prescribed by your physician.

Contents

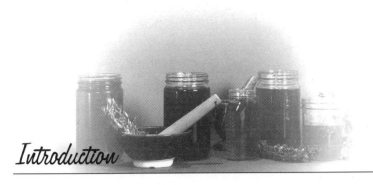

Introduction

*C*ave paintings in Spain, dating from 7000 B.C., depict men collecting honey from a bee colony. The medicinal properties of honey have been known since ancient times. A Sumerian tablet, possibly dated 3000 B.C., prescribes honey to treat an infected skin ulcer. Papyrus writings dating around 2000 B.C. from Egypt prescribe honey to treat a gaping wound of the eyebrow, penetrating to the bone:

> *Now after thou hath stitched it, thou shouldst bind fresh meat upon it, the first day. If thou findst that the stitching of the wound is loose, draw it together with two strips and thou shouldst treat it with grease and honey every day until he recovers.*

The ancient Egyptians, Assyrians, Chinese, Greeks and Romans used honey to treat a variety of ailments. Around 350 B.C., Aristotle wrote about honey being used to treat wounds and sore eyes. Muhammad, the Muslim prophet, recommended honey to treat diarrhea, and the Koran mentions the curative properties of honey. Muhammad is quoted as saying "Honey is a remedy for every illness, and the *Koran* is a remedy for all illnesses of the mind, therefore I recommend to you both remedies, the *Koran* and honey."

It should not be surprising that honey came to be used as a medicine. Transport yourself back 4,000 years and picture one of our early ancestors suffering from an open wound. How would he have eased his pain? What was available? Mud would have been the most widely available substance, and no doubt was used extensively. Mud is still used today, although scientific studies on its therapeutic benefits are few and far between. What else? What about honey—why not try it? It couldn't hurt; it might even help. Lo and behold, that sticky stuff worked a lot better than mud!

Once the therapeutic value of honey was discovered, this gift from nature–or God–was widely used to treat a variety of ailments. Ancient cultures accepted and made extensive use of this gift. The medicinal benefits of honey were passed on from generation to generation, and today honey is a popular medicine in all parts of the world, with the notable exception of the United States.

Why not the U.S.? One reason is our relatively short history with the honeybee. The honeybee is not native to the U.S., but was introduced to the East Coast in 1622 when a few hives were transported across the Atlantic; it took years for these first few colonies to expand their numbers to the point where significant quantities of honey could be harvested. It wasn't until 1853 that hives were taken to California and then onto other western states.

Perhaps if the Native Americans had the opportunity to discover honey's medicinal properties, as did natives in other countries, there would be more use of honey as a medicine in the U.S. today. European and other countries have a long and rich history of honey and honeybees and of tales of the medicinal benefits of honey. This likely explains why almost all the scientific studies on the use of honey as a medicine are in journals from outside this country. Many in the American medical community still look at honey as well outside the mainstream of medicine and are reluctant to even experiment with it for fear of being ostracized by their peers.

Another reason honey hasn't caught on as a medicine in today's U.S. is based in the psyche of our country. The Protestant work ethic–the harder you work, the further you'll advance–is woven deeply into our national fabric, along with a residual Puritan streak.

This "no free lunch" or "no pain, no gain" philosophy turns us into skeptics when something comes along that looks too good to be true. How could a great tasting food like honey be a medicine? We all know, from the time we were toddlers, that medicine doesn't taste good, that the more bitter the medicine, the more likely it is to be beneficial. Honey as a medicine flies in the face of our ingrained belief system. This book provides a rational, scientific basis for the use of honey as a medicine. This book shows that honey, in spite of its great taste, is also a remarkable medicine.

That most of the reports on honey as a medicine originate outside the U.S. has been detrimental to accepting honey as a medicine here. One of America's greatest strengths—our self-confidence, our self-esteem—can cause myopia when we view reports from other countries. There is a thin line between high self-esteem and arrogance, and too often Americans don't give proper credit to studies that were not done within our borders. Many of us have already forgotten that perhaps the two greatest scientific discoveries of the 20th century were not made by Americans: Albert Einstein, the author of the Theory of Relativity, was born in Germany; and the Englishman Francis Crick, solved the puzzle of DNA (along with American co-worker, James Watson). Our world leadership in nuclear and space technology is built upon a foundation laid by European refugees, whose own work was in turn built on earlier European studies. Readers of this book should resist the temptation to dismiss the foreign studies described here, but should objectively analyze the original references and ask themselves: "If an American had done this, would I accept it?"

In 1938 Dr. Bodog Beck (1870-1941), a physician at St. Marks Hospital in New York, published the book *Honey and Health* (Robert McBride, NY). Dr. Beck, a native of Hungary, was trained in the country of his birth and worked in a number of surgical hospitals throughout Europe before emigrating to the U.S. He brought his love of honey and his knowledge of its medicinal powers with him to the U.S., and his passion for honey permeates every page of his book. His frustration at honey not being accepted by the U.S. medical community simmers throughout his book, surfacing on occasion.

Like Beck, many European immigrants to the U.S. brought with them a knowledge of honey, and honey has been used as a folk medicine for years in the U.S., especially to relieve coughs and colds. The popular 1958 book, *Folk Medicine* by Dr. D. C. Jarvis, based mainly on anecdotes, rekindled an interest in honey as a health food in the U.S., but that interest has waned in recent years and in today's "show me the data" world, many question the use of honey as medicine.

The purpose of this book is to acquaint readers with the vast amount of solid information on the medicinal benefits of honey that has come forth in recent years. Where I've included anecdotes, one or more scientific studies are usually given to support the anecdote. In spite of the skepticism that is often directed their way, anecdotes should not be ignored. Many positive scientific studies have been initiated on the basis of anecdotal claims. Also, if you accumulate enough anecdotes, you have data. Or, as one person put it, data is the plural of anecdote.

The book is divided into four parts: Part One discusses honey's medicinal benefits; Part Two is a short section on honey for athletes; and Part Three supplies information on how to enjoy honey; finally, I include detailed information on my sources: Chapter Notes document points made in the text, followed by a bibliography of Peter Molan's sources, and a section on other sources and Web sites.

✪

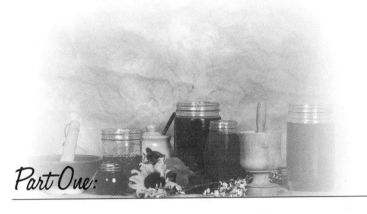

HONEY AS MEDICINE

COMPOSITION OF NECTAR AND HONEY

Composition of nectar

Nectar, from flowers, is the foundation of honey. Nectar has a much higher moisture content, or is much more watery, than honey. After bringing nectar into the hive, bees fan the nectar with their wings to evaporate most of the water, producing a more stable product with a much higher sugar content. Bees also add enzymes to nectar to produce the final product, honey, that is quite different from the original nectar.

After water, sugar is the main component of nectar. The sugar content of nectar ranges from 5% to 60%. Bees, as one might guess, prefer flower sources that contain nectar with a high sugar concentration and only work flowers with low-sugar nectar when no other options are available.

The main sugars in nectar are sucrose, glucose and fructose, while the main sugars in honey are glucose and fructose. Many nectars have a high sucrose content; bees use the enzyme invertase to convert sucrose to glucose and fructose. This conversion gives a more stable final product.

Honeybees also add the enzyme glucose oxidase to nectar. This important enzyme oxidizes, or reacts with, small amounts of glucose to produce gluconic acid, which in turn lowers the pH, increasing the acidity of the resulting honey. This lower pH stabilizes the honey, making it resistant to fermentation. This conversion of small amounts of glucose to gluconic acid produces small amounts of hydrogen peroxide as a by-product. The combination of a very low moisture content, low pH, and hydrogen peroxide not only makes honey resistant to spoilage, which is caused by microbes, but accounts for much of honey's antibacterial properties.

Composition of honey

USDA scientist Jonathan White, Jr. (1916 - 2001) worked with honey for years, and along with his colleagues, was the source for much of what we know today about the composition of honey. The following table represents the work of White and his coworkers.

AVERAGE COMPOSITION OF HONEY
(all values % except for pH)

COMPONENT	AVERAGE	RANGE
Moisture	17.2%	12.2-22.9%
Fructose	38.4	30.9-44.3
Glucose	30.3	22.9-40.7
Sucrose	1.3	0.2- 7.6
Maltose	7.3	2.7-16.0
Higher sugars	1.4	0.1- 3.8
Acid as Gluconic	0.57	0.17-1.17
Ash	0.169	0.02-1.03
Nitrogen	0.041	0.00-0.13
pH	3.91	3.42-6.10

Data from 490 samples of U.S. honey; from J.W. White's chapter in Honey, *Eva Crane, Ed. Heinemann, London 1975.*

The wide range of values for each component is due to the wide range found in the 490 floral sources used to compile this table. The different combinations of these components account for the distinctly different flavors among honeys.

Vitamins and minerals in honey

Although vitamins and minerals can be found in honey, they occur in such minute amounts that their contribution to our daily requirement is negligible. Some honey enthusiasts have greatly overstated the value of honey's vitamin and mineral content. Some people feel that these small amounts of vitamins and minerals, along with the amino acids in honey, aid in healing because they are similar to levels found in serum, but this has yet to be proven.

Microbes in honey

Although microbes can't grow in honey, microbes and their spores can be found in honey, just as they can be found in any raw food products. Microbes and their spores are ubiquitous and it would be unusual, if not impossible, to find any food product free of microbes in nature.

Botulism spores have been found in honey, just as they have been found in other food products. Botulism spores only produce damaging toxins when they grow, and they cannot grow in honey. Our immune systems can handle any botulism spores that would normally be encountered in any food products, but it takes 12 months for the immune system of infants to develop fully; therefore, neither honey nor any other raw food should ever be given to infants under the age of a year. For more information, see the chapter, "Honey for Infants."

Gamma irradiation has been shown to inactivate botulism spores and other spores in honey without affecting honey's antibacterial properties. Gamma irradiation is used to kill microbes in other food products and should gain wider acceptance in the future for use with honey. It is a safe, clean method of rendering food products safe.

Microbes in honey used as medicine should not cause concern: of more than 470 cases where unsterilized honey was used to treat open wounds, there were no reports of infection.

Other substances in honey

Honey also contains minute amounts of amino acids, protein, lipids, various enzymes and other constituents. There have been efforts, so far unsuccessful, to measure levels of some of these other components to distinguish pure honey from adulterated honey, e.g., honey to which corn syrup has been added.

IRRADIATION OF HONEY

The majority of reputable honey companies in the U.S. monitor the honey they purchase for the presence of microbes. It is very unusual for honey to have a high microbe content, but it can happen.

The possibility of introducing microbes into a sterile situation via honey is theoretically possible, but there have been no reports of this to date.

To totally eliminate the possibility of microbes in honey, producers can irradiate their product with gamma rays generated from cobalt-60. Botulism spores are one of the most difficult of all bacterial spores to eliminate, yet a 1995 study showed that 50 grams of honey spiked with 10 million botulism spores could be sterilized with a 25 kilogray (kGy) dose of gamma rays. Five thousand spores per 50 grams of honey is the upper limit of natural contamination, and at these levels 18 kGy did the job. The antibacterial properties of honey were not affected by the higher dose of radiation.

The FDA has set an upper limit of 30 kGy for irradiation of dried spices and dehydrated vegetables. More work needs to be done on setting an upper limit for honey.

The terms "irradiation" and "cobalt-60" are disconcerting to some, but there is no evidence that irradiation is hazardous to health; quite the contrary—by killing bacteria, irradiation renders food safer. For example, lives can be saved by irradiating hamburger meat to kill E. coli bacteria. Irradiation has the approval of the Food and Drug Administration, the World Health Organization, the

American Medical Society, the U.S. Dept. of Health and Human Services, the U.S. Public Service and a number of other organizations. NASA has fed its astronauts irradiated food for years.

Even Julia Child is an enthusiastic fan of irradiation, stating that "A lot of nervous Nellies are afraid of it, but there's absolutely no scientific proof that any radiation stays in the food. It just kills all the bacteria and makes the food safer."

If there are any concerns about microbes in honey, gamma irradiation should ease them. Again, evidence to date indicates that such irradiation has no effect on the antibacterial properties of honey. Irradiation is an economical procedure that adds little to the overall cost. Some grocery stores sell irradiated food products at the same price as nonirradiated. Some stores have educated their customers to pay a premium price for irradiated food, the premium being for a safer product with a longer shelf life.

HONEY AS MEDICINE

The slight regard at this time paid to the medicinal virtues of Honey, is an instance of neglect men shew to common objects, whatever their value: acting in contempt, as it were, of the immediate hand of providence, which has in general made those things most frequent, which have the greatest uses; and for that reason, we seek from the remotest part of the world, medicines of harsh and violent operation for our relief in several disorders, under which we should never suffer, if we would use what the Bee collects for us at our doors.

John Hill, M.D. (England, 1759)

That honey should have medicinal properties should not come as a surprise—honey is, after all, derived directly from the nectar of plants, and plants have been renowned for their medicinal value, both in ancient times and today. For example, digitalis and taxol provide two of our better known plant-derived pharmaceuticals. The current concern over rainforest destruction is, in good part, concern over the loss of plant species that have potential medicinal value.

That plants and nectar from plants should have medicinal value is not just a fortuitous happenstance. In order for a plant species to survive, it has had to acquire, over eons, properties that render the plant immune from, or at least resistant to, attack from microbes, as well as from insects and animals. Honeybees enhance these pre-existing medicinal properties of plant nectar by adding beneficial enzymes to the nectar and condensing it into a form—honey—that maintains its medicinal properties for prolonged periods of time.

Imagine a world without honey and without honeybees. Imagine that scientists in this world discover that plant nectars have important curative properties that are enhanced when certain enzymes are added. Now imagine how much time and effort it would take for scientists to extract the nectar from plants: micropipettes, or ultra-thin straws, could be used to suck the nectar from flowers; or flowers could be harvested, placed in a centrifuge, the nectar spun out, and then collected and filtered. The moisture content of the collected nectar would have to be reduced, by heating or evaporation, from 60% to 16% to prevent fermentation, followed by the addition of the necessary enzymes. This whole process would be so time and labor intensive that only a wealthy few could afford the finished product.

Now add honeybees to this world. The honeybee's tongue serves as a micropipette. Under the best conditions, an individual bee can make over 1,000 flower visits to collect a quarter of a teaspoon of nectar in one day. The vast number of these winged workers would not only collect significant quantities of nectar but would also lower the moisture content of the nectar to 16% (by fanning their wings to evaporate the water from the nectar). These same bees would add the necessary enzymes and produce the finished product—honey—at a cost of around one dollar per pound, wholesale. Quite a feat when you think about it! And quite a bargain when the cost of honey is compared to the cost of other plant-derived medicines. Honey is cheap because the bulk of the work is done by nonunion workers that require no benefits, other than a roof over their heads. Honey is also affordable because there is no patent on the final product. On the negative side, or from a labor management standpoint, bees refuse to work during inclement weather and, in temperate climates, bees insist on taking the entire winter off.

The medicinal benefits of honey have been attributed to its antibacterial and antifungal properties. Honey keeps well for years without refrigeration, while jams, jellies and other foods spoil in a matter of weeks. Obviously, honey has an inhibiting effect on bacteria and fungi, but it was not until the 1930s that this effect could be scientifically demonstrated.

The classic method of determining the antimicrobial properties of a substance is simple: culture a specific bacterium, or fungus, on an agar medium in a petri dish; add a test material, then see if the microbe growth is inhibited. The degree of inhibition is determined by the clear zone surrounding the introduced test substance. The antimicrobial properties of penicillin were discovered by this process in the 1930s. It is little known that, using the same test, honey has demonstrated similar antimicrobial properties.

Over the past 60 years, the inhibitory effects of honey have been tested and proven on a number of bacterial species, including many that cause human ailments. Honey has also been shown to have an inhibitory effect on a number of fungal species, including *Aspergillus flavus, A. fumigatus, A. niger, A. parasiticus, Candida albicans, C. pseudotropicalis, C reukaufil, C. stellatodidea, C. tropicalis, C. utilis, Penicillium* sp. and *Saccharomyces* sp. (from the same Molan reference as cited above).

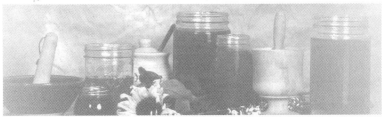

DISEASES SUCCESSFULLY TREATED WITH HONEY

Pathogen	Infection caused
Bacillus anthracis	anthrax
Corynebacterium diphtheriae	diphtheria
Escherichia coli	diarrhea, septicemia, urinary tract infections, wound infections
Haemophilus influenzae	ear infections, meningitis, respiratory infections, sinusitis
Listeria monocytogenes	meningitis
Mycobactyerium tuberculosis	tuberculosis
Pasteurella multocida	infected animal bites
Proteus species	septicemia, urinary tract infections, wound infections
Pseudomonas aeruginosa	urinary tract infections, wound infections
Salmonella species	diarrhea
Salmonella cholerae-suis	septicemia
Salmonella typhi	typhoid
Salmonella typhimurium	wound infections
Serratia marcescens	septicemia, wound infections
Shigella species	dysentery
Staphylococcus aureus	abscesses, boils, carbuncles, impetigo, wound infections
Streptococcus faecalis	urinary tract infections
Streptococcus mutans	tooth decay
Streptococcus pneumoniae	ear infections, meningitis, pneumonia, sinusitis
Streptococcus pyogenes	ear infections, impetigo, puerperal fever, rheumatic fever, scarlet fever, sore throat, wound infections
Vibrio cholerae	cholera

Note: From Peter Molan's 1992 review "The antibacterial activity of honey,
Part 1, The nature of the antibacterial activity" Bee World 73(1):5-28.
Note: since this list was published in 1992, other honey-sensitive bacteria have been reported,
most notably, Helicobacter pylori.

A number of studies showing the medicinal benefits of honey have been published in recent years. New Zealand scientist Peter Molan has done an outstanding job of summarizing many of these studies in several reviews. Molan pieced together reports from a variety of scientific and medical journals and other sources and added them up to a mountain of hard scientific data (see Molan's Mountain for a complete list of Molan's sources). The combined weight of all these studies provides indisputable proof to even the most hardened skeptic of the medicinal value of honey. Molan's work has taken honey out of the realm of folklore and placed it firmly in the realm of medicine.

In 1989, 230 years after Dr. Hill's remarks (that opened this chapter), an editorial in the *Journal of the Royal Society of Medicine* noted the impressive amount of solid work showing the medicinal benefits of honey, and stated:

> *The therapeutic potential of uncontaminated, pure honey is grossly underutilized. It is widely available in most communities and although the mechanism of action of its properties remains obscure and needs further investigation, the time has come for conventional medicine to lift the blinds off this traditional remedy and give it its due recognition.*

This 1989 editorial in a respected English journal could well have been the catalyst for the significant number of honey-medicine studies in the 1990s, including Molan's. Dr. Hill would be pleased. That virtually none of these studies took place in the U.S. indicates that the above editorial fell on deaf ears or blind eyes here.

ANTIBACTERIAL PROPERTIES OF HONEY

Four main characteristics of honey are responsible for its antibacterial properties:
1. Osmolarity
2. Acidity
3. Hydrogen peroxide production
4. Floral nectar component

Osmolarity

Honey is a supersaturated sugar solution, and as such, it has a high osmolarity. The high osmolarity of honey kills bacteria and fungi by drawing water from their cells. The water in bacterial cells seeks to come into equilibrium with the surrounding environment, and thus the bacteria and fungi are killed by dehydration. It has been shown that saturated sugar solutions have the same effect, and indeed, such solutions are used to treat burns and wounds. Sugar solution, however, lacks the three other antibacterial components.

Acidity (pH)

The scale used to measure the acidity of a substance is called pH. A pH of 7.0 is neutral, above 7 is alkaline, below 7 is acid. Values on the pH scale are logarithmic: a solution with a pH of 6 is 10 times as acidic as a solution with a pH of 7. Honey has a pH of around 4, and is therefore acidic. This acidity inhibits the growth of most bacteria.

Hydrogen peroxide production

The hydrogen peroxide producing capacity of honey, *not* its hydrogen peroxide content, is thought by many to be the main reason for honey's antibacterial activity.

Hydrogen peroxide (H_2O_2) can kill bacteria on contact and has been widely used for that purpose. Straight H_2O_2, however, is unstable and rapidly loses its effectiveness when exposed to air and light; it can also damage tissue when used in high concentrations. For these reasons, the use of pure H_2O_2 has fallen out of favor with doctors and in hospitals.

Honey has the necessary components to produce miniscule amounts of H_2O_2 over a prolonged period of time. This slow-release capability makes honey an ideal substance to use in the treatment of wounds and bacteria-caused disorders. The slow-release mechanism is a simple, chemical reaction that works as follows:

Honey is approximately 30% glucose. A much smaller component of honey is glucose oxidase, an enzyme found in the digestive system of honeybees and secreted into nectar by the bees. Under the right conditions, glucose oxidase has the ability to break down glucose into gluconic acid and hydrogen peroxide. This chemical reaction can be written as:

$$C_6H_{12}O_6 + H_2O + O_2 \rightarrow H_2O_2 + C_6H_{12}O_7$$

glucose + water + oxygen become hydrogen peroxide + gluconic acid

Honey itself, however, does not supply the right conditions for this reaction to occur.

To become active and begin breaking down the glucose in honey, the glucose oxidase requires an optimum pH of 6.1, with good activity from pH 5.5 to 8.0. The pH of undiluted honey is 3.2 to 4.5, far too low to activate the enzyme. A second condition is also required before the glucose oxidase becomes active. For the enzyme to break glucose down into hydrogen peroxide and gluconic acid, a minimum of 2300 ppm of sodium must be present. Honey has a sodium content of only 20 to 40 ppm. Therefore, pure honey stored in clean containers is stable with no reactions occurring and no H_2O_2 being produced.

But, skin and body fluids have relatively high pH and sodium levels. When honey comes in contact with skin or an open wound, the high pH and sodium levels activate the glucose oxidase and it begins to break down the glucose, releasing hydrogen peroxide — but only at the point of contact where the pH and sodium levels are optimum for the glucose oxidase to function.

To summarize, when honey comes in contact with human skin or wounds, the dormant enzyme—glucose oxidase—becomes highly active at the interface of the honey and skin or wound, as bodily fluids raise both the pH and the sodium concentration to the optimum range of enzyme activity. Thus, minute doses of hydrogen peroxide are continually released from the honey, directly to where they are most needed.

Could man devise a more perfect, slow-release antimicrobial product for treating wounds? If a billion dollar, biomedical company gave their research and development scientists unlimited time and resources, it is doubtful they could equal what nature has already provided in honey. It's enough to make even the most skeptical scientist believe in a higher being, as if God, in His wisdom, provided man with a perfect natural elixir to treat wounds and infections. Doctors in the U.S., with rare exceptions, have rejected this gift.

Floral nectar component

As one might expect, honeys vary in their medicinal effectiveness, depending on the floral source of the honey. Some honeys are more effective than others—Manuka honey from New Zealand is exceptionally effective and commands a premium price for this reason. The antibacterial variation among nectars and the honeys made from the various nectars has been explained in two ways:

1. Some nectar contains catalase, an enzyme that neutralizes hydrogen peroxide. This diminishes the effectiveness of the H_2O_2-producing mechanism of honey.

2. Some nectars contain as yet unknown substances with antibacterial properties.

Flavonoids, which are beneficial substances produced by plants, are also found in honey and are felt by some to contribute to honey's antibacterial properties. Also, honey from different flower sources has different antioxidant capacities.

In summary, the combination of osmolarity, acidity and hydrogen peroxide production makes honey a unique and powerful antibacterial agent. As if that weren't enough, additional floral components work to enhance the amazing antimicrobial properties found in some honey.

OTHER HEALTH BENEFITS

Besides its antibacterial effect, honey improves health in other ways.

Enhances the immune system

Honey can stimulate B-lymphocytes and T-lymphocytes to multiply, thus boosting the immune system.

Reduces inflammation

Honey has anti-inflammatory properties independent of its properties that combat bacterial infection. Inflammation has been reduced by honey when there were no infections involved.

Stimulates cell growth

When wounds that show no signs of healing for a long period of time are treated with honey, the healing process, and cell regeneration, begins.

Antioxidant activity

Fourteen different honeys gave varying degrees of antioxidant activity in one study. Of the 14 honeys tested, buckwheat from Illinois had the highest antioxidant content and registered 20 times higher than that of the honey with the lowest antioxidant content, sage honey from California.

Interestingly, the three honeys with the highest antioxidant content—Illinois buckwheat, California sunflower and Hawaii Christmas berry—are dark colored honeys. These are not considered high-quality eating honeys (although the strong flavor of buckwheat honey is prized by some). The three honeys with the lowest antioxidant content are all light colored, fine-quality honeys. Maybe there is something to the idea that if something tastes exceptionally good, it might not be as good for you, although antioxidant activity is only one of honey's many medicinal components.

Recent tests in New Zealand showed that Manuka honey has a very high antioxidant activity.

HONEY FOR WOUNDS

There to make a healing balsam,
From the herbs of tender fibre,
From the healing plants and flowers
From the stalks secreting honey,
From the roots, and leaves, and blossoms.

From the Kaleval (ancient Finnish tale)

To remind the reader, the sources for all the anecdotes and medical studies in this chapter and the rest of the book can be found in the Chapter Notes section at the end of the book. So that you may more easily locate a particular reference, each source is listed with its chapter name and page number.

Anecdotes

Bulgarian soldiers suffered numerous casualties while fighting the Serbian army during the Balkan War of 1913. The Bulgarians had run out of medicine to treat the wounded, but came across a small amount of honey in a nearby village. There was not enough honey to provide nourishment for the troops, but the officer in charge, a veterinarian in civilian life, decided to apply the honey to some of the wounds, not so much because he thought it would help, but to show his soldiers he cared for their welfare. A few days later, the honey-treated wounds were clean and healing rapidly while the nontreated wounds showed no improvement and had become badly infected.

"War invalid S., aged 25, had a big scar on the back of his right foot. In the center of the scar was an ulcer three by three centimetres with a deep glossy, greyish bottom and necrotic thickened edges. The patient said the wound had been in this state for three months. The application of Vishnevsky ointment, phototherapy and other methods gave no effect. Twenty days after the honey ointment was applied the ulcer healed."

After a patient's stomach incision became chronically infected and would not heal, a hospital surgeon poured honey into the wound, sutured it shut and the patient had no more problems. The surgeon was subsequently censured by the hospital's peer review committee for using this unorthodox treatment.

A severe case of meningococcal septicemia necessitated amputating both legs of a 15-year-old boy. The wounds failed to heal and were found to be infected with several species of bacteria. Standard dressings didn't help, and were painful to change. Honey was tried as a last resort. The patient recounted:

> *I can't even begin to explain how painful it was just to have a small piece of dressing changed. The nurses tried everything to make it easier, like changing the dressing in the bath, but it was agony. And it got worse. They gave me a mixture of nitrous oxide and oxygen, but towards the end that didn't work either. I felt like they were ripping my skin off.*
>
> *The nurse, Ms. Dunford, was called in because she was a specialist. Nothing was really working, so she went away to think about it and came back with the idea of using honey. She put the honey dressing on one leg and some other type of dressing on the other to compare them, but it was obvious to me really quickly that the honey was doing the job.*
>
> *For a start, the dressing didn't stick as badly, but one of the main things I noticed was that the smell wasn't nearly as bad. I'm not saying that it was worse than the pain, because the pain was bad, but the smell was one of the things that bothered me most.*
>
> *As soon as we started using the honey, the smell improved. In fact, the whole thing was easier. They were still giving me the oxygen mixture and using the bath, but it was much less painful, especially when I started listening to my own music, mainly rap and drum and bass, when they were doing it. It took a time, but eventually the nurses said, "Haven't you got anything else? People usually like to listen to relaxing music."*

Later, as reported by nurse Cheryl Dunford (MSc), "Within 10 weeks of the start of the treatment [with honey], all lesions, including the pressure ulcer, had healed completely."

This last story is from a medical report and falls in the realm between anecdote and science—you decide where it lies.

Science

For treatment of burst abdominal wounds, following cesarean delivery, 15 patients had their wounds dressed with honey and then closed with adhesive tape; the 15 patients were released two to seven days after treatment. In a separate group of 19 patients, the wounds were treated with antiseptics and resutured; the latter group was not released until nine to 18 days after treatment.

In several other different studies, honey started the healing process in nonhealing leg and diabetic ulcers that had shown no signs of healing for anywhere from six months to five years.

A 1998 study reported on nine infants that had large, open, infected wounds that did not respond to 14 days of conventional treatment. A honey dressing was applied and marked improvement was seen after five days; after 21 days of honey application, the wounds were closed, clean and sterile.

In a 1994 study, a patient with multiple ulcers on both legs had one leg treated with honey, the other received a standard treatment of fibrinolysin and calcium alginate dressing. The leg treated with honey healed much more rapidly.

In addition to the preceding studies, Molan gives scientific references for a number of other instances in which wounds have been successfully treated with honey. These include:

abrasions	a fistula
amputations	foot ulcers in lepers
abscesses	infected wounds arising from trauma
bed sores	large septic wounds
cancrum	leg ulcers
cervical ulcers	malignant ulcers
chilblains	sickle cell ulcers

cracked nipples	skin ulcers
cuts	surgical wounds
diabetic foot ulcers	wounds to the abdominal wall
perineum	other diabetic ulcers
varicose ulcers	

Why honey is a superior wound dressing

Wounds dressed with honey heal faster than with dry dressings (and some moist dressings) because there is little or no tearing of newly grown tissue when dressings are changed. Most wounds heal best in a moist environment, yet a moist environment is conducive to bacterial growth. The antibacterial properties of honey solve this Catch-22 dilemma, making honey superior to other dressings.

Using honey as a dressing

The stickiness of honey has likely discouraged many from treating wounds with honey—who wants to deal with all that stickiness? Once they try it though, most nurses and doctors find working with honey is not that difficult. Gauze or cotton pads, impregnated with honey, are available in Australia and New Zealand and are used extensively in those countries. The honey used on these pads has standardized levels of antibacterial activity and has been sterilized by gamma irradiation.

Anyone can treat wounds with honey by following these easy steps:

1. Abscesses, cavities and depressions in the wound should be filled with honey before any dressing is applied.
2. Add one ounce of honey to a 4-inch square dressing pad and apply to the wound.
3. Apply a secondary dry dressing pad on top of the honey pad, then use adhesive tape to hold both dressings in place.
4. Change dressings at least once a day (more frequently if much exudate is produced). Once the wound has stopped producing exudate, dressings can be changed once a week.

Tubes of irradiated honey are available from New Zealand and are more convenient, but plain honey from a jar can be used. Although there are no known reports of problems with honey that has not been irradiated, using irradiated honey is preferred.

Just as all honeys are not equal in their medicinal value, all Manuka honeys are not equal. Peter Molan introduced the Unique Manuka Factor (UMF) to rate the antibacterial potency of a given honey. The UMF is determined by comparing the antibacterial activity of a given honey with the antibacterial activity of antiseptic phenol (carbolic) using a standard lab test. A UMF rating of 4 is equivalent to the potency of a 4% solution of phenol, a rating of 10 is equivalent to a 10% phenol solution. See Molan's web site at http://honey.bio.waikato.ac.nz for further information.

Medical professionals in New Zealand use Manuka honey with a UMF rating of 10 or higher. If buying Manuka honey for medicinal purposes, check the label for a UMF rating. Tests are currently being conducted on a number of different U.S. honeys to determine their antibacterial potency. Results of this testing can be followed on the Honey Board web site, at www.honey.com.

✪

Honey with a high UMF rating is more costly. For example, a 17 ounce jar of honey with a UMF rating of 10 or better is available at www.manukahoneyusa.com or (800) 395-2196 for $25, as of this printing. A single 17 oz. jar of nonrated Manuka honey sells for $3.39 at Trader Joes (2001 prices).

Honey's antibacterial and physical properties make it ideal for treating wounds. Wounds treated with honey not only heal faster, but there is less scarring after healing. In 2000, the use of honey in wound treatment was succinctly summarized by a respected U.S. physician: "Honey as a topical antibiotic agent has several efficient properties: it is natural, the risk of allergy is low, it has a broad antibacterial spectrum without the risk of resistance, and it is quite economical."

HONEY FOR BURNS

Anecdotes

A man suffered severe burns when boiling water spilled on his hand; he treated the hand with honey, except for his thumb, which did not appear to be badly burned. The following day, the hand was still red, but blisters were absent, while the thumb was heavily blistered. Continued treatment with honey led to rapid healing.

In another instance, a registered nurse suffered a burn on one arm and applied a commercial burn ointment. A week or so later, she received a similar burn on the other arm and applied honey. A few weeks later, the honey-treated arm was completely healed; the ointment-treated burn was still evident.

Science

There are three widely used methods to treat burns: silver sulfadizine, polyurethane film and amniotic membrane. Dr. M. Subrahmanyam compared honey treatment with these three methods in three separate studies in the 1990s.

In the first study, 104 burn victims were divided into two groups of 52 patients. One group received the conventional treatment (silver sulfadizine), the other group was treated with honey. Within seven days, 91% of the wounds treated with honey were free from infection, compared to less than 7% using conventional treatment. Within 15 days, 87% of the honey-treated wounds were healed versus 10% with the conventional treatment.

In the second study, two groups of 46 burn victims had their wounds dressed with honey. The victims healed in a mean time of 10.8 days compared to 15.3 days for victims treated with polyurethane film (OpSite). Twice as many of the polyurethane-dressed wounds became infected compared to the honey treatment.

In the third study, 46 burn patients treated with honey-impregnated gauze had their burns healed in a mean time of 9.4 days compared to 17.5 days for 24 patients treated with amniotic membrane.

There were residual scars in 8% of the patients treated with honey versus 16.6% of those treated with amniotic membrane.

A respected scientist with the Biomedical Research Foundation in Maastricht, The Netherlands, reviewed the effects of honey on burns and concluded:

> *Burns that are treated with honey heal more rapidly and effectively in a patient-friendly way, without infection complications, and with little pain and relatively little scarring. The honey-treated burns enter their end phase within six weeks, which is unique and not seen with any other wound dressing. Honey treatment of burns is certainly cost effective because it shortens the duration of treatment by about 25% and it certainly reduces the rate of hospitalization. The rediscovery of honey in this millennium and its registration as a medical device will turn a 5,000-year-old folk remedy into a clinically accepted wound dressing of today.*

Shouldn't honey, preferably gamma irradiated, be on hand at all burn units in the United States?

HONEY FOR STOMACH PROBLEMS

Ulcer anecdotes

There are numerous anecdotes of honey's effectiveness in treating ulcers. These anecdotes date back well before a bacterium was found to be the main cause of ulcers (in the 1980s). Three anecdotes are given below:

A man suffering from severe, possibly terminal stomach ulcers, hated doctors, so he stayed home and suffered. A friend told him about a Russian study showing that honey cured ulcers. The man embarked on a honey diet—honey and freshly squeezed grapefruit juice, nothing else—and was miraculously cured.

In his 1938 book, *Honey and Health* Dr. Bodog Beck states:

Dr. Schacht, of Wiesbaden, Germany, claims to have cured many hope-less cases of gastric and intestinal ulcers with honey and without opera-tions. It is rather unusual that a physician of standing has the courage and conviction to praise honey. The beekeepers and their friends know that honey will cure gastric and intestinal ulcerations, this distressing and most dangerous malady, a precursor of cancer. But the news has not yet reached 99% of the medical profession. The remaining few physicians who know it, are afraid to suggest such an unscientific and plebian rem-edy, for fear of being laughed at by their colleagues.

A number of Russian studies in the 1940s and 1950s showed that honey could cure ulcers. In one study, out of 302 patients with ulcers, normal treatment gave a healing rate of 29%, and honey gave a healing rate of 59.2%. The honey treatment also gave a general tonic effect: increased weight, improved gastric acidity and blood composition; plus, a tranquilizing effect on the nervous system was observed, with patients becoming calm and more cheerful.

Science

Stomach ulcers have been shown to be caused mainly by the *Helicobacter pylori* bacterium. There is also a solid link between *H. pylori* and stomach cancer. Honey inhibits *H. pylori*.

Researchers at Hebrew University of Jerusalem, in Israel, proved that taking two to three ounces of honey everyday for several months wipes out the toughest-to-treat ulcers.

It is possible that another mechanism other than its antibacteri-al properties is responsible for honey's effectiveness against ulcers. It has been shown that honey can stimulate sensory nerves in the stomach. These are the same nerves that respond to capsaicin, the irritant in chili peppers, causing the release of selective peptides which increase the blood supply to the stomach, which in turn helps protect the stomach lining from damage.

Diarrhea, irritable bowel syndrome, etc. anecdotes

There are numerous anecdotes that regular honey consumption relieves diarrhea, irritable bowel syndrome (IBS) and other gastrointestinal disorders, and that honey consumption leads to normal, regular bowel movements. The Russian, N. Yoirish, reported on a study by a Professor M. Golumb, in which honey was the prescribed treatment for toxic-infectious diarrhea in children. Golumb found that the course of the disease was less severe and recovery came more quickly with honey, and the children receiving honey put on two and a half times more weight than the children that didn't receive honey.

Science

In general, antibiotics give a dramatic improvement in irritable bowel syndrome, indicating a microbial cause, but symptoms usually return in a few months, thus showing that antibiotics are not a long-term solution to IBS.

In a test with two groups of patients suffering from diarrhea caused by bacterial gastroenteritis, those that were treated with honey had a mean recovery time of 58 hours compared with 93 hours for the other group.

Evidence is mounting that bacteria cause most stomach and gastrointestinal problems. There are also indications that stomach problems caused by bacteria are a precursor to stomach cancer. Antibiotics, which can kill all intestinal flora, both good and bad, may not be the best solution. Certainly more studies should be undertaken to confirm or disprove anecdotal tales on the benefits of honey in treating and solving these problems.

HONEY FOR INFANTS

First, let me state unequivocally that honey is not recommended for infants under one year of age. Around 1978, researchers discovered that botulism spores can reside in honey, just as they can be found in any other raw food product. Raw foods of any kind are not recommended for infants. It takes a year for the immune system of infants to develop, and neither honey nor any other raw food should be given to infants less than 12 months old. On many honey containers, the label reads, "Do not feed to infants under one year of age." I have no quarrel with that statement.

Now, please follow me to the end of this chapter—there's a good punch line waiting there.

First, let's look at why honey was a popular infant supplement prior to 1978. In a 1938 study on infant feeding, doctors found that honey was absorbed into the bloodstream more quickly than any other sugar except straight glucose, yet honey did not flood the bloodstream with an overabundance of sugar that could not be handled by the body. The authors of the study stated, "In view of the fact that honey is a product ready for use without artificial treatment and that it is composed of [the] two sugars most acceptable to the body, it is strange that it has not enjoyed wider use, especially in the feeding of infants."

As a result of this study, and by word of mouth, many mothers added or continued to add honey to baby bottles, and some pediatricians recommended the practice for infants, including those less than 12 months old. There is also evidence that honey can raise the hemoglobin content of children's blood, with beneficial results.

During the year that it takes for their immune systems to develop, infants are very vulnerable to a wide range of diseases and infections. Prior to antibiotics, infant death rates were considerably higher than they are today. Bacterial infections played a major role in this higher infant mortality.

Now, consider a recent U.S. study implicating the bacteria *Helicobacter pylori* in sudden infant death syndrome (SIDS). Yes, this is the same bacteria that is the major cause of stomach ulcers, and one that some consider the most widespread bacterium involved in chronic infections. Researchers found that 28 out of 32 SIDS infants had been infected with *H. pylori*, compared to only one of eight non-SIDS babies who had died of other causes.

Here we have a bacterium implicated as a pernicious baby killer, and an agent—honey—known to suppress that killer, but not recommended for all infants. What to do? The answer is simple: gamma irradiate the honey. If pediatricians do not recommend honey for infants under one year of age because their immune systems are not sufficiently developed, shouldn't pediatricians recommend *gamma-irradiated* honey for all infants for the exact same reason? In fact, in light of *H. pylori's* implication in SIDS and honey's effectiveness against *H. pylori*, shouldn't all pediatricians seriously consider prescribing gamma-irradiated honey for infants?

Now ponder this question: if *H. pylori* bacteria are indeed a major cause of SIDS (and one study does not prove this), would the number of deaths from SIDS over the past 20 years caused by not feeding infants honey have exceeded the number of deaths from botulism if those infants were fed honey? And, has the incidence of SIDS increased since mothers stopped putting honey in their baby's bottle?

The honey industry is missing a good bet by not placing gamma-irradiated honey in the baby section of supermarkets. Until that day comes, concerned mothers should consider gamma irradiating their own honey. Most metropolitan areas have gamma irradiation facilities, as do many clinics and hospitals.

HONEY FOR THE EYES

I have cured a Horse stone blind with Honey

and Salt and a little crock of a pot mixed.

In less than three daies, it hath eaten off

a tough filme, and the Horse never complained after.

Vigerius

Anecdotes

In 350 B.C., Aristotle wrote that "White honey is a good salve for sore eyes." In India, lotus honey is said to be a panacea for eye diseases. The ancient Mayan compilation, *Pharmacopoeia*, mentions honey as a cure for cataracts. The honey was from stingless bees, not honeybees, as there were no honeybees in ancient Mexico. However, the healing properties of both honeys should be similar. Commercial honey eyedrops are sold today in Mexico as well as in Brazil and Venezuela.

N. Yoirish, the Russian, stated, "On the advice of Professor E. Fisher of the Ophthalmology Department of the Odessa Regional Clinical Hospital, Ukraine, honey ointments are widely used for various lesions of the cornea." Yoirish goes on to claim that honey gave a marked improvement in patients suffering from severe keratitis, or inflammation of the cornea, after conventional treatments failed.

In 1937, a beekeeper gave credence to the chapter's opening quote from Vigerius when he wrote to a bee journal: "I had a horse going blind with a white film over his eye which seemed to hurt. His eye was shut and watered. I dipped white honey into his eye with a feather for several nights. In a day or so the film was gone and the eye looked bright and good."

In the 1930s, 40s and 50s, a Dr. Carey practiced medicine in Southern California, and was known for clearing up cases of cataracts with honey, as follows: a drop of honey in each eye at night before going to bed, which may sting a bit at first; then wash the eyes out in the morning. Cary felt part of the healing effect was due to honey drawing out fluid from behind the eye. Cary related the story of how a California woman who couldn't see to thread a needle or read a newspaper was told by her ophthalmologist that she had cataracts, but that he wouldn't operate until they got bigger. She decided to treat her eyes with honey, and within three weeks she could thread a needle and read the paper. When she returned to her ophthalmologist two months later, he could not see any evidence of the cataracts.

Science

After conventional treatment failed, 102 patients with a variety of eye disorders, such as keratitis, conjunctivitis, blepharitis etc., were treated with honey. The honey was applied under the lower eyelid as any eye ointment would be applied. Improvement was seen in 85% of the cases, with no deterioration in the condition of the patients in the other 15%.

Blindness in half of the roughly 26 million blind people in the world is caused by cataracts, a defect of the lens of the eye. Apparently, honey has properties that allow it to penetrate to the well-protected lens. One researcher speculates that flavonoids present in honey have the necessary properties to access the lens. Antioxidant and osmotic properties of honey could also be a factor. Certainly the potential benefits of honey to treat cataracts deserves more study.

HONEY FOR THE SKIN

Honey, and honey mixed with other substances, serves as a skin conditioner for many people around the world. The antibacterial properties of honey protect and rejuvenate the skin. According to Janice Cox, author of *Natural Beauty at Home* "Honey's antimicrobial properties make it useful for the treatment of minor acne flare-ups. Also, unlike some acne treatments, honey doesn't dry the skin."

Honey is a good all-purpose skin conditioner, and far cheaper than the expensive creams and lotions found in cosmetic departments. The National Honey Board gives the following home recipes for skin and hair treatment with honey:

For the Skin
Skin-softening bath
Add 1/4 cup honey to bath water for a fragrant, silky bath.

Smoothing skin lotion

Mix 1 teaspoon honey with 1 teaspoon vegetable oil and 1/4 teaspoon lemon juice. Rub into hands, elbows, heels and anywhere that feels dry. Leave on 10 minutes. Rinse off with water.

Moisture mask

Mix 2 tablespoons honey with 2 tablespoons milk. Smooth over face and throat. Leave on 10 minutes. Rinse off with warm water.

Honey cleansing scrub

Mix 1 tablespoon honey with 2 tablespoons finely ground almonds and 1/2 teaspoon lemon juice. Rub gently onto face. Rinse with warm water.

Firming face mask

Mix together 1 tablespoon honey, 1 egg white, 1 teaspoon glycerin (available at drug and beauty stores), and enough flour to form a paste. Smooth over face and throat. Leave on 10 minutes. Wash off with warm water.

Facial toner

In a blender, puree 1 tablespoon honey with a peeled, cored apple. Smooth over face. Leave on 15 minutes. Rinse with cool water.

Smoothing skin clarifier (for minor, acne flare-ups)

Mix ½ cup warm water with ¼ teaspoon salt. Using a cotton ball, apply directly to blemish. Maintain pressure with cotton ball for several minutes to soften blemish. Using a cotton swab, dab honey on blemish; leave on 10 minutes. Rinse and pat dry.

For the Hair

Hair conditioner

Mix ½ cup honey with ¼ cup olive oil. (Use 2 tablespoons oil for normal to oily hair). Work a small amount at a time through hair until coated. Cover hair with a shower cap; leave on 30 minutes.

Remove shower cap; shampoo well and rinse. Dry as normal.

Hair shine

Stir 1 teaspoon honey into 4 cups (1 quart) warm water. (Blondes may wish to add a squeeze of lemon). After shampooing, pour mixture through hair. Do not rinse out. Dry as normal.

HONEY FOR OTHER MALADIES

Hangovers

The relatively high fructose content of honey and its enzyme content speed the metabolism of alcohol and give quicker recovery from overindulgence.

Cramps, tics and twitches

Cramps and the nervous twitching of facial muscles, such as eyelids, the corners of the mouth and other muscles, can be eliminated by taking two teaspoonfuls of honey at each meal. Honey contains acetylcholine which acts as a chemical transmitter of nerve impulses.

Coughs, colds and flu

Honey is still widely used in this country as a folk remedy for coughs, colds, and flu. There are reams of anecdotes on the benefits of honey for these ailments, but no scientific studies.

Here's some food for thought. The great flu epidemic of 1918 killed 20 million worldwide, including 500,000 Americans. It would be helpful to know what percentage of those that perished were honey eaters compared to the general population.

Have you stocked up on honey for the next flu epidemic?

Liver Problems

Glucose, a major component of honey, increases glycogen

stores in the liver. Glycogen, in turn, amplifies the liver's ability to filter and neutralize bacterial toxins. There are no scientific studies on honey's effect on the liver. For now, three anecdotes (all from the same source) will have to suffice:

> *Patient S. contracted hepatitis in 1922. Owing to extreme weakness, frequent vomiting and pain in the region of the liver, he was confined to bed, put on a severe diet, and given medication. There was no improvement so he decided to try honey and was soon cured of jaundice; the pain ceased and he has been well ever since.*

> *Patient L., who had been suffering from cholelithiasis and cholecystitis for a long time, freed himself from unbearable pains by eating honey regularly.*

> *Patient A. suffered from hepatitis and was cured of it by eating honey.*

Dental Health and Strokes

The oft quoted homily "sugar rots your teeth" should be amended, for accuracy, to "sucrose rots your teeth; honey is good for teeth." Tooth decay requires sucrose to form plaque. Table sugar is 100% sucrose, while honey is mostly glucose and fructose. In addition, the antibacterial properties of honey help fight tooth decay.

Bacteria from the mouth can enter the bloodstream and increase plaque in the arteries, which in turn can trigger strokes by impeding the flow of blood to the brain. Researchers at the University of Buffalo have shown that people with severe gum disease have a doubled risk of strokes.

Honey and Cancer

There are reports that honey both inhibits and kills cancer cells and can prevent the spread or metastasis of cancer. The World Health Organization (WHO) has classified *Helicobacter pylori*, the bacterium that causes most stomach ulcers, as a Class 1 carcinogen. *H. pylori* is strongly linked with stomach cancer.

When surgery is used to remove cancer, recurrence of tumors at the surgery site is a concern. In a 2000 study, 60 mice were divided into two groups of 30 each, and each group was inoculated with tumors. Group A mice formed the control group, Group B mice had their wounds coated with honey before and after inoculation. Tumor implantation occurred in only eight out of the 30 honey-treated mice versus 30 out of 30 in the control group. Dr. Tonia Young-Farok, a Mayo Clinic surgeon, feels substances in honey might actually help dissolve tumor cells, and stated, "It's not clear what the power of honey is, but there's certainly something here that's of interest."

In their 1965 annual report, the New York Cancer Research Institute stated that "Beekeepers have the lowest incidence of cancer of all the occupations." However, a 1979 study obtained death certificates of 580 beekeepers and found that beekeepers "had only a slightly lower than expected fraction of deaths from cancer" compared to the general population. The study was initiated to prove that bee venom had no effect on cancer. Bee venom is thought by some to increase cancer due to a build-up of antigens in the bloodstream over a period of prolonged exposure to bee stings. The study did not consider the potential anticarcinogenic properties of honey, and honey is barely mentioned in the study. It is possible that the inhibitory effects of honey on cancer cancelled out the harmful effects of a high antigen load in the bloodstream. Unfortunately, the authors did not address this point.

Miscellaneous Problems

Other maladies for which there is currently only anecdotal information on the benefits of honey include athlete's foot, bed wetting (the moisture absorbing capacity of honey is felt to play a role here), arthritis, hay fever and insomnia.

Hay fever caused by pollen is felt by some to be curable, or at least reduced in severity, by consuming local honey. The theory is that the few pollen grains that wind up in honey induce a degree of resistance to hay fever when the honey is consumed. I'm a bit skeptical of this, but some people really believe it.

Honey was used as a contraceptive in ancient times; an Egyptian prescription used powdered crocodile feces or elephant dung, saltpeter and honey. Cotton, soaked in honey and lemon juice, is allegedly used as a contraceptive in Egypt today. Recent work in New Zealand showed that honey kills sperm. Besides being a spermicide, topical application of honey should also act as barrier against sexually transmitted diseases (STDs) and possibly as a treatment for such diseases.

In Alzheimer's Disease, the brain loses 90% of its acetylcholine, a neurotransmitter used by cells in areas of the brain that are most important for memory formation. Honey is a good source of acetylcholine. My business has put me in contact with hundreds of beekeepers over the years, and none that I know of have developed Alzheimer's. I know many beekeepers who are mentally sharp well into their eighties and nineties.

DO GERMS CAUSE ALL AILMENTS?

A growing body of evidence implicates germs in a number of medical problems. The first breakthrough in this line of thinking occurred in 1982 when an Australian researcher, Barry Marshall, proposed and then proved that a bacterium was the main cause of stomach ulcers. Many in the medical community scoffed when these reports first came out. Everyone knew that stress was the cause of ulcers and treatment of the symptoms, not the cause, was based on this "fact." It should be noted that this was the same medical community that accepted bloodletting as the preferred remedy for a number of ailments a couple of centuries ago, and that routinely overprescribes antibiotics today. Today, ulcers are typically treated with antibiotics and, by an informed few, with honey.

Recently, the same bacteria that causes ulcers (*H. pylori*) has been implicated in sudden death syndrome, or SIDS. Some feel that *H. pylori* is the most chronic infection in the world.

Bacteria have recently been implicated in both heart disease and in adult-onset asthma. The bacterium *Chlamydia pneumoniae* has been strongly associated with people that have had heart attacks. Doctors at Boston University compared the records of 16,000 British patients and found that those that had taken antibiotics were only one-third to one-half as likely to have suffered heart attacks. The same bacterium, *C. pneumoniae*, along with another, *Mycoplasma pneumoniae* have been found in lung biopsies taken from asthmatics; antibiotics curbed the asthma.

In 2000, Amherst College biology professor, Paul Ewald, published the book *Plague Time: How Stealth Infections Cause Cancers, Heart Disease and Other Deadly Ailments*. Ewald maintains that microbes are responsible for virtually all human ailments. His book is looked at with skepticism by many in the medical community. But if only half of it is verified in coming years, it will force a change in how we look at human health.

As bacteria are implicated in more and more ailments, honey, with its antibacterial properties, should assume a greater role in our daily lives.

HONEY: A REMEDY FOR ANTIBIOTIC RESISTANCE

There have been recurring articles in recent years on the growing resistance of many germs to antibiotics. Penicillin is no longer effective against a number of pathogens. Vancomycin, developed in 1958, has long been considered the best weapon against bacteria no longer vulnerable to other drugs, but it, too, is losing its effectiveness. Almost every human infection—including malaria, tuberculosis, gonorrhea, pneumonia, even leprosy—is now resistant to at least one major class of antibiotics, according to experts, and the situation can only get worse.

Honey's mode of action in suppressing microbes is far different and more natural than that of antibiotics, and therefore, germ resistance is less likely with honey. Most microbes need moisture to sustain life and it would seem difficult for microbes to develop resistance to the moisture-extracting properties of honey. Much of honey's antimicrobial activity is bacteriostatic (freezing the bacteria in time and preventing them from spreading) rather than bactericidal, or killing the bacteria. Resistance by bacteria is more likely to arise to an agent that kills them, as is the case with most antibiotics, because the few surviving bacteria (and there are always a few) pass on their resistant genes to future generations. To date, no resistance of pathogens to honey has been reported, although admittedly, unlike antibiotics, honey has not been used widely enough to say that some mode of resistance could not develop.

There is general agreement that antibiotics are overprescribed. This overuse of antibiotics is due in part to patients demanding an easy fix, and to drug companies promoting that easy fix. Many of today's antibiotics are indiscriminate killers. When taken by mouth, they kill all the flora in the gastrointestinal tract, both good and bad. Such indiscriminate killing can throw the whole system off balance, according to gastroenterologist John O. Hunter of Addenbrooke's Hospital in Cambridge, England. Our bodies contain beneficial microbes, and these microbes are less affected by honey than they are by most antibiotics.

Certainly, the medical community, and informed individuals, should take a close look at honey as an alternative to antibiotics in the treatment of many common maladies. There is evidence that after a prolonged period of not coming into contact with a particular antibiotic, germs can lose their resistance to that particular antibiotic. Antibiotics should be seen as the treatment of last resort, rather then the first quick fix. The use of honey for minor maladies will prolong the effectiveness of antibiotics for major ailments.

Honey for Hospitals

In recent years, hospitals have developed a reputation for being reservoirs for resistant forms of the *Staphylococcus aureus* bacteria, otherwise known as staph. Staph is now resistant to penicillin and is becoming resistant to vancomycin, which has replaced penicillin as an antibiotic in many situations. Spending time in a hospital, particularly when surgery is concerned, can be hazardous to your health because of the proliferation of antibiotic-resistant staph bacteria in hospitals.

Considering that *Staphylococcus aureus* is one of the species of bacteria that is most suppressed by honey, shouldn't all hospitals have gamma-irradiated honey in their cafeterias and on the menu for all hospital meals, plus being ever present in the operating room?

When planning a hospital stay, it might be wise to pack a jar or two of honey.

HONEY: A MEDICINE WITHOUT A PROFIT

Imagine seeing a jar of honey with the label shown on the opposite page.

Now, substitute Versitol® or a similar name for honey and put "I.C. Pharmaceuticals, Inc." at the bottom of the label.

Can you envision a multimillion-dollar advertising campaign for Versitol, with ads appearing nightly on your TV screen, depicting charts of test results and satisfied users of Versitol? Can you see I.C. Pharmaceutical representatives swarming doctors' offices, leaving free samples along with reams of literature on the benefits of Versitol?

Most drug companies look at one standardized test showing positive results for a product and see big dollar signs. They parade the results of the test over and over, milking it until it is more than dry. Imagine what a drug company would do with the scores of

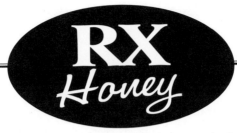

Honey has been shown to provide relief for, or to cure, a number of different disorders, including, but not limited to the following:

Diarrhea, ulcers, infections, irritable bowel syndrome (IBS), gastrointestinal problems, cancer and staphylococcus (staph) infections.

Infectious diseases caused by bacteria that are sensitive to **Honey** include the following:

Anthrax, diphtheria, urinary tract infections, ear infections, meningitis, respiratory infections, sinusitis, pneumonia, tuberculosis, infected animal bites, typhoid, dysentery, abscesses, boils, carbuncles, impetigo, tooth decay, puerperal fever, rheumatic fever, scarlet fever, sore throat and cholera.

A number of different types of wounds have been successfully treated with **Honey**, including:

abrasions, amputations, abscesses, bed sores, burns, burst abdominal wounds following cesarean delivery, cancrum, cervical ulcers, chilblains, cracked nipples, cuts, diabetic foot ulcers and other diabetic ulcers, a fistula, foot ulcers in lepers, infected wounds arising from trauma, large septic wounds, leg ulcers, malignant ulcers, sickle cell ulcers, skin ulcers, surgical wounds, wounds to the abdominal wall and perineum, varicose ulcers.

The medicinal benefits of **Honey** are due to honey's antibacterial properties and its moisture-retaining properties.

Side effects: None

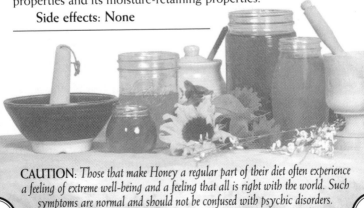

CAUTION: *Those that make Honey a regular part of their diet often experience a feeling of extreme well-being and a feeling that all is right with the world. Such symptoms are normal and should not be confused with psychic disorders.*

solid, unbiased, positive tests showing honey's clear-cut medicinal benefits. They'd have so much to work with, they wouldn't know where to start.

The cautionary statements on many current medicines run into the hundreds, even thousands of words, and reading them is like taking a walk on the dark side, yet the total sales for many of these products are well into the millions of dollars. Imagine how much a product like Versitol would make for a company. What salesman wouldn't jump at the chance to sell Versitol?

Large pharmaceutical companies haven't entered the medicinal honey market because honey is not a proprietary product—anyone can bottle and sell honey. Drug companies are being shortsighted here; as discussed, all types of honey have medicinal benefits, but some, such as Manuka, are significantly better than others. Coming up with a standardized, microbe-free (via gamma irradiation), high-activity medicinal honey—a given dose of which would provide the same benefits time after time after time—could well be a very profitable venture for a drug company.

There are, in fact, such medicinal honey products being produced by companies in several other countries. Medi-Honey, based in Australia, sells sterilized honey in both tubes and jars. You can find their products on their web site at www.medihoney.com/index.htm. Comvita in New Zealand also sells tubes and jars of honey for medicinal purposes. Their web site is www.comvita.com/contact.htm.

Both the above companies use Manuka honey from New Zealand as the main honey in their products because of Manuka's proven antibacterial potency. Several European companies sell medicinal honey and a number of South American countries sell honey eyedrops. We may see the day when plants that produce nectar with a high medicinal value are cultivated by farmers solely for their nectar and subsequent honey. Look for some Manuka plantings in the U.S. in the future.

One company retails a 60 gram tube (a little over two ounces) of Manuka honey for $8.98 and a one pound jar for $6.49. With the wholesale price of honey at less than a dollar a pound, there is obviously a profit in selling medicinal honey.

Certainly, some work must be done to produce a uniform, commercial medicinal honey, but it is just because of this that there is an enormous opportunity for a U.S. drug company, or entrepreneur, to capitalize on the vast potential market for such a product. The product would have to be sterilized, probably by gamma radiation, as most current products are, but this is a relatively simple and economical process.

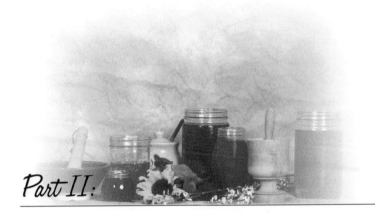

Part II:

HONEY FOR ATHLETES

THE ULTIMATE SPORTS DRINK

Most athletes, including weekend athletes, have heard that taking honey before a race or a game improves performance. Honey is superior to sugar in this regard because honey's two main components, glucose and fructose, act as a one-two punch to provide energy. The body uses glucose immediately, while fructose must be converted to glucose in order to be metabolized; thus, the fructose acts as a slow-release energy source. Sugar, on the other hand, is solely sucrose, readily available as an energy source, but without any backup.

Since their introduction in the early 1980s, sports drinks such as Gatorade® have become very popular in America. Gatorade sales worldwide hit $2.1 billion in 2000. By comparison, sales of U.S. honey have held at less than $200 million for the past 20 years. Gatorade is a product of the Quaker Oats Company and accounted for approximately 40% of Quaker's total sales and operating income. Gatorade holds about an 85% share of the U.S. sports drink market. PepsiCo bought out Quaker Oats in 2001, probably for the sole purpose of acquiring Gatorade.

Sports drinks or power drinks contain a mixture of sucrose, glucose and fructose as their energy source. Water, obviously, is the main ingredient in sports drinks: they are usually well over 90% H_2O. The most popular sports drink contains roughly one half pound of sugar per gallon. One half pint of honey (0.7 lbs) would provide this same half pound of sugars. Sports drinks also contain small amounts of sodium and potassium (about one tenth of an ounce per gallon) to replenish and maintain the body's mineral and electrolyte levels that are lost to perspiration.

One gallon of sports drink sells for about $4.00; one half pint of honey generally costs one or two dollars. Obviously, honey is a much cheaper energy source than the pure sugar energy source of sports drinks. Athletes could use honey, water and a sodium-potassium pill and be as well off, if not better off, than athletes using sports drinks.

Some sports drink makers claim that the balance or mix of sugars in their product is better (the term "scientifically formulated" is sometimes used), but there is little or no evidence to support this claim. The main sugar in the most popular sports drink, Gatorade, is sucrose. The main sugar in the recently introduced Powerade (a subsidiary of Coca Cola) is fructose from high-fructose corn syrup. Apparently these two companies don't agree on which sugar is best. Because the sports drink market is so lucrative, it's certainly possible that we'll see a honey-based sports drink in coming years.

Realizing that a major cost of sports drinks is transporting water around the country, drink manufacturers also sell a dehydrated product to which water must be added, although the final cost is not much different than buying the liquid mix. Dehydrated honey can also be purchased, although the market and outlets are limited.

Anecdotal tales on the benefits of honey to athletes are also supported by science. A 1955 report showed that athletes participating in endurance tests showed better performance when fed two tablespoonfuls of honey 30 minutes prior to the test. Tests included repeated running of 50-yard sprints, continuous running at a rate of one mile in six minutes and repeatedly swimming 100-yard distances.

A National Honey Board release (April 4, 2001) reported the results of a test in which nine competitive cyclists used honey to improve endurance. Compared to a placebo, honey cut three minutes off their time to complete a 40-mile race and produced 6% greater cycling power.

Another study funded by the Honey Board and reported by CBS HealthWatch (6/23/01) stated:

Previous studies have shown that the combination of carbohydrates and protein supplements are beneficial to boosting muscle recovery, but they did not look at what types of carbohydrates. Using honey as the carbohydrate source, researchers found that when it is combined with a protein supplement, subjects maintained better glucose levels, or blood sugar levels, which is an important part of post-workout recovery.

"The beneficial thing with honey is that it helped maintain glucose levels positively after two hours of workout," says Dr. Richard Kreider, lead author of the study and director of the Exercise and Sport Nutrition Laboratory at the University of Memphis, Tennessee.

Other sports nutritionists say it is heartening to know that something as inexpensive as honey can perform as equally well as some of the pricey supplements on the market, including maltodexrin and Endurox.

"The name of the game is recovery," says Susan Kleiner, PhD, RD, and owner of High Performance Nutrition, a sports nutrition and consulting firm in Seattle, Washington. "Honey is affordable and widely available. To know that it works for recovery is good news for everyone who is fitness minded."

Until a honey-based sports drink becomes available, why not save money by using honey mixed with water and a couple of sodium-potassium pills?

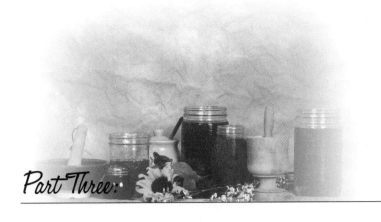

Part Three

THE JOY OF HONEY
かる
LA JOIE DU MIEL

KINDS OF HONEY

"Pick up a jar of honey on your way home from work, honey."

Although the above statement might be heard, the proper rejoinder, "What kind?" is rarely made, and the shopper usually opts for the cheapest honey available. Big mistake!

As with any commodity, the cheapest is usually the poorest quality, and honey is no different. Beekeepers use the expression "crankcase oil" to describe poor quality honey, and though some of this poor quality honey sits on store shelves, much of it goes to the bakery trade where its flavor is greatly diluted and little noticed. Often, it is packed in cans rather than jars to disguise its less than attractive appearance.

Few shoppers would buy rotten produce, even at a heavy discount. Unfortunately, one can't detect quality differences in honey by looks or by reading the label. Tasting is the only sure method, and this is not allowed in most stores. Once the cheapest honey finds a place on the kitchen table, it is rarely used for the simple reason that it doesn't taste good. What a shame! The consumer misses out on a potential gastronomical treat, and the honey industry loses a potential customer.

Other potential honey consumers are turned off by the small, opaque packets of honey served in restaurants and on airlines. These businesses watch their bottom line carefully and usually opt for the cheapest honey available, often because they are unaware of the wide variation in honey quality. The diner that tries honey from these packets, if not turned off by the taste, too often finds it unremarkable. Again, the diner misses out on a rewarding honey experience and honey producers lose a potential customer.

People should be aware of the wide variety of honeys available: every floral source (and there are thousands of floral sources from which bees make honey) produces a distinct flavor of honey. Although a few different floral sources of honey can be found on store shelves, most store-bought honey is a blend from different sources. As a general rule, light-colored honey tastes better and is milder than darker honey. Buckwheat honey, a dark honey, is an exception; its strong flavor is prized by some, though disliked by others.

Because honeybees often work a variety of flower sources, it is sometimes difficult to get a true unifloral honey. Clover honey and orange honey are exceptions because they are grown in a monoculture environment; their flowers bloom in abundance with few plants offering competing blossoms. Some honey packers blend a superior honey with an inferior one to achieve a palatable end product (some wine makers do the same), although there is a recent trend toward selling quality honey at a premium price. The highest priced honey in the store is usually the best. Sioux Honey, a beekeeper cooperative, does a god job on quality control. Other commercial packers also take pride in their product, and do a good job. Experiment with different brands and flower sources to find one you like. High-quality honey can be purchased directly from a beekeeper or at a farmers' market. Ask questions of a beekeeper about quality, and you'll usually get a straight, and sometimes lengthy, answer.

Over a thousand of the many thousands of honey flavors are described in the book *American Honey Plants*. Sixty-one popular American honeys taken from that book are listed here. The next chapter covers 18 superior or gourmet honeys, 15 of which are taken from this list, with the remaining three originating beyond our country's borders.

POPULAR AMERICAN HONEYS		
Alder	Fiddleneck	**Orange**
Alfalfa	**Fireweed**	
Anise	Foxglove	Palmetto
Asparagus	Fuchsia	Peppermint
Aster		
Avocado	Gallberry	Rabbit brush
	Goldenrod	Rape
Basswood		Raspberry
Bay tree	**Heather**	
Bird foot trefoil	Holly	**Sage**
Blackberry	Horehound	Sainfoin
Blueberry	Hyssop	Salt cedar
Blue curl		Sassafras
Buckwheat	Knapweed	Saw palmetto
		Sourwood
Cactus, giant	Larkspur	**Star thistle**
Canola	Lima bean	Sunflower
Cantaloupe		
Carrot	**Macadamia**	Tamarisk
Clematis	Magnolia	**Thyme**
Clover	Manzanita	**Tupelo**
Cotton	Meadow foam	
Cranberry	**Mesquite**	Vetch
	Mint	
Eucalyptus	M. Monroe	Wildflower

Note: Bold type indicates superior quality honey. All but one of the above were condensed from a list of over 1,000 American honey plants described in American Honey Plants *by Frank C. Pellett. Dadant & Sons, Hamilton, Illinois (1947) (3rd printing 1978)*

The discerning reader will notice "Saw palmetto" on the accompanying list of honey flavors and will be aware that Saw palmetto is sold as an herb—it is felt to reduce the likelihood of prostate cancer. Saw palmetto (and Saw palmetto honey) is found in the Gulf Coast region, and it is not unreasonable to believe that Saw palmetto honey would retain many of the properties of the plant.

At the local supermarket, there are entire aisles devoted to wine—different varieties, different brands, different prices (when asked to pick up a bottle of wine at the store, one usually asks "What kind?"). Unfortunately, the honey section of a supermarket is quite small, usually only a few feet wide, because consumers are not yet honey-wise; there are no weekly honey columns in the local newspaper, nor magazines devoted entirely to honey. It is up to consumers to educate themselves about honey; trial and error is the best method. Start by exploring www.honey.com.

SUPERIOR AND GOURMET HONEYS

Many who have been introduced to the different flavors of honey are hooked for life, always trying new flavors to experience a different taste sensation. Because of the virtually infinite number of flavors available, this is a never-ending quest. As with life, the journey is more rewarding than the destination because of the stops along the way. With the modern-day addition to honey of fruit flavors, such as raspberry, the number of taste combinations multiplies.

Honey connoisseurs have sung the praises of honey since ancient times. For good reason "Nectar of the gods" is a well-worn phrase. One passionate honey aficionado assembled his collection, Midas-like, and waxed eloquent:

> It's difficult to appreciate the subtle and minute differences in honey until you actually see several hundred bottles, of several hundred varieties, all together in rows and stacks and groups. If you have seen a display such as this you know what I mean. If not, you have a life event yet to experience.

Flavors? Every jar of honey has its own flavor. Minty. Cloying. Sweet, but a tangy aftertaste. Sharp. Strong, but a mild aftertaste. Metallic. Definitely citrus. Fruity. Bold. Sugary, but smooth. Nearly tasteless, but a sharp aftertaste. Molasses-like. The list goes on and on and on.

I've had friends over, not aware of these differences, and had them sample five or 10, 15 or 20 different kinds of honey. Their awakening is a joy to watch. The sugar buzz they get is almost frightening, however. If you try this I suggest moderation in amount, and in number, or not. It's fun either way.

I've always wanted to get together a group of wine tasters, connoisseurs if you will, and give them several varieties of honey to try. "Rich bouquet," "fine nose," "good body," glowing aftertaste," all these fine wine words would apply equally well here. Can't you just hear one of those famous wine critics? "Yes, a nearly pure sourwood, perhaps 1993 or 1994 from northeast South Carolina or southeast North Carolina. Heated to, oh, no more than 120 degrees, strained, but not filtered, and definitely not blended. Not the best year for sourwood, 1995 was better, a bit lighter and without the smoky aftertaste. But this wasn't a bad year either. Probably from a smaller producer and hand extracted and bottled. Maybe stored in a freezer for a bit since it hasn't darkened much. A bit of waxy feel on the back of the tongue perhaps, which adds to its rustic appeal."

The wine analogy is apt, and has been used by a number of honey lovers. Honey devotees can be just as passionate, or annoying, as wine connoisseurs.

We have stores in the U.S. that sell nothing but wine, but few that sell nothing but honey, and those that do usually have a limited selection. Not surprisingly, the French are much more aware of honey flavors than we are. Listen, as another honey aficionado tells of his visit to a honey store in Paris:

One of the highlights of our trip was a visit to the Parisian store La Maison du Miel, roughly translated as "The House of Honey." I hap-

pened to read of its existence in a guidebook, and immediately insisted to my wife that we cross town on a rainy day to visit. I was intrigued that an entire store would exist that sold nothing but honey and honey products, and curious about how the food-crazy French would approach selling honey in the sophisticated Paris market.

The store is on a small street [24 rue Vignon] near the famous Louvre art museum, and its business card advertises it as selling "honey from all the provinces, the most beautiful varieties and the best price." It also notes that the store is fairly new by French standards; founded in 1898, it [has just passed] its one-century anniversary. When I entered the store, the first thing to catch my eye was a beautiful tiled bee inlaid on the floor, looking very much like murals we had seen in restored ruins from the ancient Roman occupation of France. The next thing that caught my eye was the bar. No, they didn't serve alcohol, but they did serve honey from all regions of France and a few other places around the world. The storekeeper was positioned behind the bar, handing out elegant, small silver spoons which customers could dip into any of the open honey jars on the counter for tasting.

The honeys were almost all from France, labeled with floral sources, and the distinctive color and flavor of each honey made it obvious that great care had been taken to keep the honeys unifloral. They were organized by regions, with dark and light honeys arrayed in no particular order, including a small section at the end for non-French honey. Sorry, Americans, but U.S. honeys were not to be found in this store, although they did have the ever popular Canadian clover and buckwheat honeys, some extremely dark Turkish honey that looked more like strong coffee than honey, acacia honey from Hungary, and a honey that was scantily described only as "honey from Greece." Each honey was labeled as sauvage or culture, indicating whether it came from natural vegetation or from a crop.

My personal favorite was the lavender honey, produced in the region of southern France where I spoke to the beekeepers. This honey comes from the bright purple flowers of lavender plants raised to produce oils used in perfumes, and had a highly distinctive, lightly aromatic taste. I closed my *eyes as I savored my spoonful of this ambrosial honey, with images of beautiful French models wearing high-fashion clothing dancing across my palate.*

Flower sources are abundant in cities and one or more residents often has a colony or two of honeybees. City bees produce interesting honeys because of the wide variety of available flowers (about as far from monoculture as one can get). Open a jar of honey you have brought back from a faraway city and memories of that city will come flooding back as the scent and taste embrace you. There are over 100 bee colonies in Paris, some of them housed at the jardin de Luxembourg in Paris' sixth district. The jardin holds an annual honey sale each autumn, and in recent years this "Honey Day" has included a beekeeping demonstration.

For the discriminating honey buyer, 18 honeys that are generally considered of superior or gourmet quality are listed on page 49 and 50; fifteen are from the United States and three are from overseas. I've tried only about half the honeys on this list. My personal favorites (with an admittedly western U.S. bias) are clover honey from Montana and its surrounding states, sage honey from Southern California and star thistle honey from northern California.

Prior to the time that I kept around 400 colonies of bees in the 1970s, orange honey was one of my favorites. After several years of consuming more orange honey than I care to think about, I grew tired of the flavor, but it's still a favorite of many. I come back to orange honey occasionally, and it never fails to remind me, not of idyllic hours spent with a gentle breeze wafting through fragrant orange blossoms and the musical hum of millions of happy bees accompanied by a Mozart concerto playing on the truck stereo (although there were a few such blissful moments, but I didn't have, or thought I didn't have, the time to smell the flowers during those years), but of lifting 100 pound boxes of honey in 100 degree weather in coveralls soaked with sweat while scores of angry bees registered their objection to my intrusion by inflicting numerous stings on any exposed bit of skin or pinning wet coveralls to flesh; of long nights driving a truckload of bees, then sleeping, or trying to sleep, in the cab of the truck until the bees could be unloaded at daylight; the angry buzz of unseen bees echoing in my ears as they crawled up pant legs and down collars; of twisting and turning until a moment comes when I must k—k—k—. Ah, but I digress.

Many consider California's sage honey to be one of the finest of all honeys. Noted apiculturist, A.I. Root, was taken by sage honey and expressed the following sentiments in the late 19th century:

> *I well remember the first taste I had of the mountain sage honey. Mr. Langstroth was visiting me at the time, and his exclamations were much like my own, only that he declared that it was almost identical in flavor with the famed honey of Hymettus, of which we had received a sample some years ago. Well, this honey of Hymettus, which has been celebrated in both prose and poetry for ages past, was gathered from the mountain thyme, and the botany tells us that thyme and sage are closely related.*

Although most visitors to California avoid our Central Valley (primarily because visitors generally come during the heat of summer), there is no more beautiful scene in California, or anywhere else, than orchard bloom in February and March. Almonds bloom in mid-February, producing vistas of white almond blossoms as far as the eye can see. Peaches, prunes, cherries and apples bloom after almonds and provide a similar dazzling show.

Thousands make the trek to New England each fall to view the fall colors. The equally spectacular spring colors in California's San Joaquin Valley is one of the world's best-kept secrets. Autumn colors are unquestionably beautiful, but there is also an attendant somberness as one senses the days getting shorter. In contrast, spring blossoms rejuvenate both body and soul, filling one with the sense that all things are possible. Bees and beekeepers are especially attuned to the seasons. Talk to a beekeeper in April and you'll find a buoyant optimist, and the bees will have a noticeably happy hum; talk to that same beekeeper in the fall and you may find a different person, and the bees, clustered in the hive, will have a melancholic, sometimes irritable tone.

Epicureans looking for new taste sensations would do well to track down some of the splendid honeys that are available to anyone with the perseverance to find them. It's unlikely you'll find them in the supermarket; start at www.honey.com or www.honeylocator.com.

EIGHTEEN SUPERIOR-QUALITY GOURMET HONEYS		
Name	**Where found**	**Remarks**
Acacia	Italy, France, China	Different species give different flavors
Buckwheat	Most states	Dark; strong flavor; popular in Europe
Cactus, giant	Southern Arizona	Unique because of locale; resists granulation
Clover	Northern tier states	Pure clover honey is hard to beat
Eucalyptus	CA and other states	Distinct flavor; some love it, some don't
Fireweed	Washington, Alaska	Erratic production in some areas
Heather	Scotland, Ireland	Dark, thick; distinctive flavor
Lavender	Italy, U.K., France	Granulates smoothly; popular in Europe
Macadamia	Hawaii	Prized by some; unique because of locale
Mesquite	Southwest states	Granulates easily; flavor can vary annually

Orange	Calif., Florida	Distinct flavor; favored by many
Raspberry	Northern states	High quality with a raspberry taste
Sage	California	Slow to granulate; several species
Sourwood	Carolinas, E. Tenn.	Slow to granulate; prized by many
Star thistle	No. Calif., Oregon	Considered a weed by ranchers
Thyme	NE states, Greece	Praised by the ancient Romans
Tupelo	Florida; Gulf states	Featured in *Ulee's Gold* with Peter Fonda
Wildflower	All countries	Catchall name; some is great, some isn't

TOXIC HONEYS

Plants produce a variety of toxic substances as a defense against attack from insects and animals, yet instances of toxic honey are rare; poisoning of livestock by direct ingestion of the poisonous plant is far more common. When plant toxins do get into nectar, the resultant honey often has a bitter taste, making it unlikely to be consumed. Also, some toxic nectar kills the bees before they can convert it to honey.

A number of plants have been reported to produce poison honey, including mountain laurel and rhododendron. Actually, there are 29 species of rhododendron in the U.S., and the bulk of these reports concern the rhododendron family. Jimson weed and yellow jasmine have also been reported to produce poison honey.

There are anecdotal reports of toxic honey going back to ancient times. Symptoms include vomiting, diarrhea, dizziness, low blood pressure—at least one or two deaths have been reported. Uncapped, unripe honey (closer to pure nectar) from poisonous plants is far more likely to be toxic than honey that has been ripened in the hive.

It is of interest that Native Americans also made use of the same plants that produce poisonous nectar, applying a bit of poison from the plants to the tips of arrows or darts. The fact that poisonous plants also produce poisonous nectar gives credence to the idea that plants with medicinal value produce nectar with medicinal value, Manuka being a prime example.

STORING HONEY

Honey is a supersaturated solution of sugars, mainly fructose and glucose, and over time the sugar (mainly the glucose) in most honey separates out to form crystals, a process called granulation. The coarseness of the crystals gives the honey a gritty or sandy texture that is unpleasant to some, and no problems to others. The overall taste is unaffected. Also, partially granulated honey in a glass jar is visually less appealing and harder to sell than a clear, ungranulated product.

Honeys from different flower sources vary considerably in their susceptibility to granulation: sage and tupelo honey are quite resistant and remain clear for years. A few honeys are very susceptible to granulation and start to granulate within a few weeks, or in the case of canola and blue curl honey, within a few days.

The crystals in granulated honey have a reduced moisture content, therefore the moisture content of the remaining liquid portion is increased. This increase in moisture makes the liquid portion more susceptible to fermentation, although this has not proved to be a significant problem. I have consumed honey that has been partially granulated for several years that still tasted fine.

Granulated honey can be easily reliquefied by heating. Placing a jar of granulated honey in a pan of warm water usually suffices. Putting a container of granulated honey in an enclosed car on a sunny day is another method. A few years ago, I had a five gallon can of granulated honey that I liquefied by leaving it in the sauna room of a local gym overnight. Using a microwave, with due caution, is also a solution.

When heating granulated honey, temperatures should be around 100° to 160°F. Keeping the granulated honey at 145° for half an hour is a frequent recommendation; however, the temperature should never exceed 160°F. High temperature and prolonged heating can impair both the flavor and antibacterial properties of honey.

The granulation or crystallization process requires a starter particle on which crystals form and expand. For this reason, most commercial honey is filtered and strained to eliminate extraneous particles and to give a clearer final product. Honey must be heated to between 140° and 160°F in order to pass easily through filters. Commercial honey packers are careful not to overheat honey. Although filtered honey is very resistant to granulation, some consumers prefer unheated, unfiltered honey. Such honey is occasionally found in a health food store, but usually available only by direct purchase from a local beekeeper.

The granulation process can also be purposefully controlled to produce an excellent product called spun honey or whipped honey. Spun honey is a solidified honey with a creamy texture. Spun honey is honey that has completely granulated, but with extremely fine granules. The granulation process in spun honey is purposely initiated by introducing to liquid honey a few very fine, honey particles (sometimes from a previous batch of spun honey). The resulting crystals are also extremely fine, giving the final product a smooth, creamy texture. Most Canadian honey is sold as spun honey. Spun honey is an excellent product and more easily spread and less messy than regular honey. However, it is not as visually appealing as clear, regular honey, and is usually sold in opaque containers. Spun honey used to be called, and is sometime still called, cream or creme honey. This appellation has fallen out of favor because of the negative connotations of the word "cream" with health- and weight-conscious consumers. There is no difference, except for looks, between spun (or cream or whipped) honey and regular liquid honey.

The optimum temperature for honey granulation to occur is between 55° and 57°F. Storage above or below this temperature retards granulation. Storage at cooler temperatures is recommended for the best retention of honey quality. Storing in a dark place or in an opaque container reduces any harmful effects light may have on honey. There are some indications that light can reduce the antimicrobial properties of honey.

Granulation can be eliminated by storing honey at freezing temperatures (32°F). In one study, honey stored at 32°F for five weeks, then allowed to sit at 57°F, showed no granulation for two years; the same honey, without the previous cold treatment, granulated within two weeks of being stored at 57°F.

If buying honey from a local source, ask for this year's crop. Buy no more than a six-month supply at one time; keep one jar on the table, one in the cupboard, one in the medicine chest, one in the bathroom and the rest in the freezer. If you haven't done so already, try spun honey—once you try it you may decide, as many people have, to not use anything else. And then you never have to worry about granulation.

BUYING HONEY

I went to the forest to collect honey.
I went, I went, I went
I went very far, beyond the big river.
I heard the sound of bees. I saw up high the place of honey
I said, "Nobody has enclosed the tree with vine, it is mine, it is my
honey."

I sharpened my axe, very sharp indeed.
I cut a vine. I fanned my fire, and put the fire
In my basket.
I began to climb; I climbed, I climbed.
The honey was very far. It was honey, real honey, not apuma
I put fire in the hole. I blew. I got much smoke
I drove out many bees.
I chopped, I chopped, I chopped.

> *Excerpt from an African song relating a legend of natives*
> *of the Itari forest between the Congo River and Lake Albert*

In ancient times, honey was an expensive delicacy available only to a very few. It was a scarce commodity because there were no domesticated bee colonies—all honey was harvested from feral colonies, and not without great effort. In many parts of the world, honey from feral colonies is still a major source.

Today, due to modern beekeeping practices, honey is available to all strata of society at an affordable, even cheap, price. When buying honey, the shopper should have at least some background knowledge. Unfortunately, this knowledge is available only through the kind of experience gained through trial and error, not from *Consumer Reports*. Forearmed with knowledge, the consumer can make intelligent honey-buying decisions. There is currently much work going on to determine the medicinal effectiveness of various honeys. You can follow the results of this work at the Honey Board web site, www.nhb.org, or in media reports.

Because of the wide variety of flower sources, honey has a wide variety of flavors. Experiment a bit to decide on the flavor you like. Once decided, you can purchase that variety in the supermarket, if they carry it, or at your local farmers' market. You can also go online to find a seller; try going to www.honeylocator.com to see what you can find. When traveling, seek out local producers of honey. Most roadside fruit stands sell honey.

Flower sources for many of the finest honeys in the world are located right here in the U.S. and are exclusive to our country. Some of these fine honeys sell at a price slightly above the average price, but they are well worth it. It hasn't happened yet, but as people become more knowledgeable about honey, look for the day when some of these fine honeys sell at two or three times the going rate, just as fine wines do.

American beekeepers do an exceptional job of producing a superior product, and their methods and facilities for extracting and packing honey all must meet or exceed health standards that are stricter than those in most countries. Honey imported into the U.S. is generally of lower quality than U.S. honey. The United States consumes around 500 million pounds of honey annually. U.S. bee-keepers produce less than half of this amount—the rest is imported. If you want high-quality U.S. honey, ask questions of your grocer, or write letters to find out where your honey originated. Where a honey was packed is not a true indication of its origin, as most foreign honey enters the U.S. in large drums and is packed into smaller containers after it arrives here.

Some unscrupulous souls sell honey that has been blended or adulterated with cheaper sweeteners such as corn syrup. Tests can detect such substances as corn syrup and sugar in honey and most packers run these tests. New substances, called honey analogs, complicate the matter because they are more difficult to detect. To be sure you're getting pure honey, not an adulterated product, know with whom you're dealing when you buy honey.

Try to get the freshest, most recently produced honey possible. In the temperate U.S., honey purchased in the spring is usually last year's honey; honey purchased in the fall or early winter is likely to be this year's honey. To be sure, ask; you don't want to be buying two- or three-year-old honey.

Although honey can be stored for years at room temperature and still be quite palatable, there is some deterioration in flavor and in medicinal value over time. Therefore, buy no more than a six-month supply at any one time.

RECIPES

My favorite recipe:

To one cup of hot tea (or coffee) add
1 tablespoon of honey, stir well
and sip slowly.

Those that experiment with honey in place of sugar to sweeten coffee or tea rarely go back to sugar. Honey imparts a taste that enhances—or disguises—the flavor of ordinary coffees and teas and often makes superior blends even better. Different kinds of honey impart subtly different flavors to the final mixture.

For those that don't sweeten coffee or tea, honey can be substituted for sugar on cereals and for jam on toast. Probably more honey is consumed at breakfast than at any other time.

Honey can replace all the sugar in most recipes, using about 20% more honey than the amount of sugar called for to account for the moisture in honey. Start by substituting honey for half the sugar called for in a recipe. When replacing sugar with honey in recipes, also:

- Reduce the liquid (water, juice or milk) in the recipe by 1 tablespoon for each 4 tablespoons (1/4 cup) of honey used.
- Increase the amount of baking soda required by $\frac{1}{2}$ teaspoon for each cup of honey used.
- Reduce oven temperature by 25 degrees F to prevent over-browning.

Baklava and its tasty layers of flaky, honey-filled pastry is a popular pastry in Mediterranean countries and a gourmet delicacy in the U.S. The pastry layers are made from phyllo dough (available in some supermarkets and in Greek or Mediterranean grocery stores), honey, butter and one or more of the following ingredients: almonds, walnuts, pecans, eggs, cinnamon and other spices.

Honey is the major ingredient in some of the finest barbeque sauces. Sue Bee puts out an outstanding barbeque sauce that is 48% honey.

There is a myriad of honey recipe books. A recent handsome example is *Honey, A Connoisseur's Guide with Recipes* by Gene Opton and Nancy Huges, from 10 Speed Press in Berkeley, California. Most honey sellers also supply recipes. Recipes can also be obtained from the National Honey Board, 390 Lashley St., Longmont, CO 80501, (303) 776-2337, or at www.honey.com.

MEAD AND HONEY ALE

Mead

> *Fill the honey'd bev'rage high,*
> *Fill the skulls, 'tis Odin's cry!*
> *Heard ye not the powerful call,*
> *Thundering through the vaulted hall?*
> *Fill the meath and spread the board,*
> *Vassals of the grisly lord!*
> *The feast begins, the skull goes round,*
> *Laughter shouts — the shouts resound*
>
> From the *Carousal of Odin* (Penrose)

Mead is honey wine, using honey as the sugar source instead of grapes. Honey is also used in other alcoholic drinks, most notably Drambouie, Irish Mist and Polish Krupnik.

Mead was man's first fermented drink; its history can be traced to 334 B.C. Mead was eventually supplanted by wine, just as sugar has supplanted honey as the preferred sweetener. Mead was enjoyed, even worshipped, by our ancient ancestors. A number of ancient Greek and Roman writers—Plato, Plutarch, Theocritus, Pliny—mention mead in their writings. Mead is still popular with many today, as the rosters of the several mead societies in the U.S.

indicate. Mead's popularity is growing as people seek new taste sensations. In the highly competitive wine business, winemakers are looking for products that stand out from the crowd. Mead, the honey wine, certainly fits the bill.

One has to hunt to find mead in a wine or grocery store, but there are indications that this is changing. We will likely see one or more of the large winemakers get into the mead business in the coming years. Any new product that is of good quality and stands out from its shelf mates should be a winner.

Recent information that alcohol, in moderation, is good for overall health could be combined with information on the medicinal benefits of honey to market mead as a health tonic. The wine people, not the honey people, will be the ones to bottle, promote and sell mead, because the wine industry has the necessary capital to take on the task of generating a successful promotional campaign. Roger Morse (see below) suggested that Robin Hood would be an excellent character around which to build a promotional program: "C'mon, lads, lets raise one to Little John and toast today's success!"

The guru of mead was Cornell professor of apiculture, Roger Morse (1928-2000). His book *Making Mead* is the Mead bible, and is a small but comprehensive book that covers all aspects of mead and mead making.

Honey Ale

From the bonny bells of heather
They brewed a drink lang-syne,
Was sweeter far than honey,
Was stronger far than wine.

They brewed it and they drank it,
And lay in blessed sound
For days and days together
In their dwelling under ground.

Reference to heather ale in Robert Louis Stevenson's *A Galloway Legend*

Honey ale, made from the nectar of heather, has a long and interesting history. It was widely used by the Picts, a tribe of people that flourished in England from 300 to 840 A.D. When the Picts merged with the Scots, the secret of brewing heather ale was lost, because the Picts would not divulge it.

Legend has it that when the last two living members of the Pict clan, father and son, were brought to the Scot ruler, Kenneth the Conqueror, he offered them their lives in exchange for the secret of making heather ale, the properties of which were felt to impart untold strength to those that consume it. When the pair refused, the son was killed and the father imprisoned. The father lived many more years, and when blind and bedridden as an old man, he overheard some young men boasting of their strength. The old man told them they were feeble compared to men who drank heather ale; he asked for an iron bar and broke it with his hands.

Heather was noted for its medicinal properties. The treatise *Theatrum Botanicum*, 1640 A.D., had this to say about heather:

> *It hath a digesting quality, resolving the malignity of humors, by transpiration or sweating; which a decoction of the flowers being drunken, doth perform, and thereby giveth much ease to the paines within the body, and expelleth the worms therein also; the leaves and flowers made into a decoction is good against the stings or biting of serpents and other venomous creatures; and the same being drunk warm, for thirty days together, morning and evening, doth absolutely breake the stone [likely referring to stones in the bladder or kidney] and drive it forth; the same, also, of the distilled water of the whole plant, being drunke easeth the cholicke; the said water of the juyce of the herbe dropped into the eyes helpeth the weaknesse of the sight.*

So far, the market for honey ale and honey beer is limited, but we should see that market increase as microbreweries increase their share of the beer and ale market. In 2001, Sioux Honey introduced Sue Bee Honey Ale to a few Midwestern states. According to a spokesman "One of the common misconceptions is that it's a sweet beverage, and it's not. It has perhaps a touch of sweetness, but it's definitely a beer." The honey in honey ales enables the yeast to produce more alcohol, creating a light beer that is about 5% alcohol.

If interested, look for mead and honey ale or honey beer in stores or ask for it in restaurants or pubs.

OTHER PRODUCTS OF BEES

Bees produce a variety of products besides honey; you've likely heard of some of them. A short discussion of seven different products is given here. With the exception of propolis, the medicinal benefits of these products remains unproven.

Pollen

Pollen has been called the "beef steak" of the bee colony and provides more and better nutrition than does nectar. Pollen is rich in protein, minerals and vitamins. Bee-collected pollen is sold in health food stores and other outlets. There is a wide variation in the nutritional value of pollen, depending on flower source.

Propolis

Propolis is a resinous material collected from plants by bees. It is a sticky, gummy substance that bees use to seal cracks or openings in their hives. There are documented studies on the antibacterial activity of propolis. In a recent study, when scientists applied propolis to the teeth of rats, the cavity rate was reduced by 60% and production of an enzyme that encourages plaque growth was almost halted. Apparently, rats get dental cavities just as we do, so theoretically propolis should have the same salutary effect on our teeth.

As with pollen and honey, propolis derived from different plants has different characteristics, thus making it difficult to get a product with uniform medicinal properties. There is certainly enough positive information on the benefits of propolis to warrant further studies, especially to determine the medicinal value of propolis derived from different plant sources. It is likely that plants producing honey with the greatest medicinal value would also produce propolis with similar characteristics.

Besides being sold in health food stores, propolis is used as an additive to skin lotions, beauty creams, soaps, shampoos, lipsticks, chewing gum, toothpaste, mouthwashes and sunscreens.

Royal Jelly

Royal jelly is a glandular secretion of worker bees and is used as a food for queen bee larvae. Health and potency claims for royal jelly are dubious, with scant scientific support.

Venom

There are hundreds of anecdotes on the benefits of bee venom for arthritis sufferers. Unfortunately, there are no controlled studies to support the stories for humans and few to disprove them. One reputable study on arthritic dogs showed definite beneficial effects from venom injections: higher cortisol levels and significantly increased mobility.

I treated my arthritic knee with bee stings a few years back with little or no benefit, and I know a number of beekeepers that suffer from arthritis in spite of receiving numerous stings. On the other hand, I know some people, including beekeepers, who have no doubt that bee stings relieve their arthritis. The different types of arthritis and the different chemical makeup of individuals could explain why some people react differently than others, just as there are wide differences in allergic reaction to stings among individuals. The stories I've heard on the beneficial effects of bee stings for arthritis are credible, and the study on dogs is further evidence that something positive is going on. The unpleasantness of the treatment, for both doctor and patient, along with the possibility of an allergic reaction (which could trigger a lawsuit) has undoubtedly hindered tests with bee venom, but certainly this subject should be investigated further. Numerous stories demonstrate that bee venom combats, even cures, multiple sclerosis, but again, there is little or no supportive evidence.

Wax

Wax is secreted by glands in the abdomens of honeybees. Bees use this wax to build their comb nests. The biggest market for beeswax is in cosmetics, mostly for lipstick, creams, ointment and lotions. The candle industry is also a major user of beeswax, as are companies that produce waterproofing and polishing materials.

Bee brood

Bee brood, the grub-like larvae of bees, is a highly nutritious food and is considered fit for human consumption in some countries, and in certain cultures, even considered a delicacy. It's a tasty product, either raw or cooked (usually fried). When bears tear into a bee colony, they enjoy the brood as much as or more than the honey. There is no real market for bee brood in this country, most of it is sold in Asia, but things could change in the future.

Pollination

Pollination is not a tangible product of bees, but the rental of bees to pollinate a variety of crops—almonds, apples, melons, cranberries, and many more—is a major source of income for U.S. beekeepers, exceeding honey income for some. The value of bees to U.S. agriculture runs into the billions of dollars, far more than the value of the honey produced by the bees.

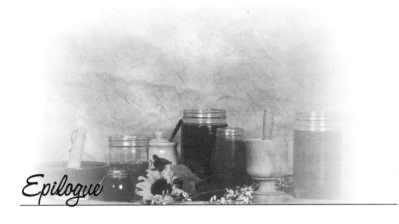

The great number of positive studies on the medicinal benefits of honey, virtually all of them from outside our borders, should encourage U.S. scientists and doctors to investigate honey more thoroughly. Certainly there needs to be more controlled scientific tests on the medicinal benefits of honey and much more work on developing a product with uniformly high antibacterial activity. Such studies will be costly and the honey industry, beleaguered by low prices because of global competition, does not have the resources to fund such tests (although, to their credit, honey producers are funding a few).

The National Institute of Health (NIH) is currently spending $14 million to evaluate the effectiveness of glucosamine to treat arthritis. Why not fund studies on the effectiveness of honey on a number of maladies? If honey became an accepted medicine in the U.S., think of the billions of dollars that could be saved—dollars that would otherwise go to prescription drugs. It's not too far-fetched to think that if honey became an accepted medicine, our economy would become more stable and our country more productive. A healthy population provides tremendous economic benefits. It has been estimated that a meager 1% reduction in the mortality rate of cancer alone would have an economic value of $500 billion to the U.S.

Play a word association game using the word "honey" with doctors around the world: the most frequently associated word for U.S. doctors might well be "botulism;" for New Zealand doctors, "medicine;" for German doctors, "health;" and for French doctors, "treat." Honey still lies well outside the mainstream of medicine in this country. Eliminating the botulism stigma from honey, which in my opinion was vastly overstated in the first place, by using only gamma-irradiated honey in medical experiments should allow U.S. medical scientists to explore honey's benefits with impunity.

My background is in horticulture, and over 20 years ago, a respected horticultural scientist encouraged his students to think outside the box. His comments are just as applicable to young medical students today:

> It is a foolish young scientist who does not soon learn that the Court of the Inquisition still sits in judgment on the unorthodox. In 1616, it forced Galileo to submit to the orthodoxy of the theologians. Today's equivalent comes from a web of bureaucratic rules and policies. All are well intentioned, but their cumulative effect is to exert a powerful pressure towards orthodoxy. Our bright young people need to be allowed a little more freedom and a chance to prove themselves original thinkers without the system whipping them into traditional, sometimes unimaginative channels.
>
> W. Grierson

Does such a climate as described exist today? You bet it does!

Witness the reaction when it was proposed by Australian Barry Marshall that the bacterium, *H. pylori*, was the main cause of ulcers. The poor man was pilloried (if not pyloried), especially in the U.S., for daring to question an accepted doctrine of the medical establishment, thereby questioning the establishment itself. Fortunately, Marshall had the stomach (and I mean *literally* had the stomach: he swallowed a solution laced with *H. pylori* to prove his point; wouldn't that make a good book or movie?) to pursue his hypothesis to a successful resolution. More recently, Paul Ewald is enduring blows for proposing that microbes cause most human ailments. The jury is still out on this one.

It is hoped that a young U.S. medical student (or future medical student) will read this book, and Peter Molan's work and other work, and, in an appropriate situation, ask his mentor "I've got a bit of honey here. Why don't we try it, just to see what happens?"

✪

Chapter Notes

INTRODUCTION

p. ix

Line 1. Eva Crane, ed., *Honey* (London: Heinemann, 1979)

Line 2-7 (plus four-line quote). Richard Jones, *Honey and Healing* (Cardiff, UK: IBRA, 2001); *Bee World* 78, no. 3 (1997): 146-149; the quote came from G. Manjo, *The Healing Hand*, (Boston: Harvard University Press, 1975).

Lines 8, 9 (after quote). P. Molan, "Why Honey is Effective as a Medicine," *Bee World* 80, no. 2, (1999): 80-92

Line 11 (Muhammad quote). Eva Crane, ed., *Honey* (London: Heinemann, 1979), p.464

PART I: HONEY AS MEDICINE

Composition of Honey and Nectar

p. 1

Last paragraph. D.M. Burgett, "The Occurrence of Glucose Oxidase in the Honeys of Social Hymenoptera," (Ph.D. dissertation, Cornell University, 1973).

See also T.D. Brock, *Biology of Organisms* (Englewood Cliffs, NJ: Prentice Hall, 1970).

p. 3

(vitamins and minerals). Eva Crane, ed., *Honey* (London: Heinemann, 1979). Table 8 from Crane's book compares the vitamin and mineral content of honey with recommended daily requirements. The serum reference is from Cheryl Dunford, "Using Honey as a Dressing for Infected Skin Lesions," *NT Plus* 96, no. 14 (Apr. 6, 2000): 7-9.

Last paragraph (microbes, 470 cases). P. Molan, "A Brief Review of Honey as a Clinical Dressing," *Primary Intention* 6, no. 4 (2001):148-158; also cited in Molan's 2001 review in *Bee World* 82, no. 1 (2001): 22-40. A thorough overall review of microbes in honey was published in 1999: Jill Snowden, "The Microbiology of Honey," *American Bee Journal* (Jan. 1999): 51-60.

Irradiation of Honey

p. 4

4th paragraph. T. Postmes et al., "The Sterilization of Honey with Cobalt-60 Gamma Radiation: a Study of Honey Spiked with Spores of Clostridium bot-

ulinum and Bacillus subtillis," *Experientia* 51 (1995): 986-989. See also P. Molan
and K. Allen, "The Effect of Gamma Irradiation on the Antibacterial Activity of
Honey," *Journal of Pharmacy and Pharmacology* 48 (1996): 1206-1209.

5th paragraph, first sentence. "Irradiation of Horticultural crops at Iowa
State University," *HortScience* 32, no. 4 (1997): 582-585.

p.5

2nd paragraph (Julia Child). "Irradiated Food—is it the Answer?" *Western
Grower and Shipper* (June 1993).

A good review of food irradiation is "Radiation Pasteurization of Food,"
Council for Agricultural Science and Technology Issue paper no. 7 (April 1996)
4420 West Lincoln Way, Ames, IA 50014

Liquids can be sterilized by high-pressure pasteurization; see Neil
Mermelstein, "High-pressure Pasteurization of Juice," *Food Technology* 53, no. 4
(April 1999): 86-90. This method has been modified for honey.

Honey As Medicine

p.5

Opening quote. Dr. John Hill, *The Virtues of Honey in Preventing Many of the
Worse Disorders; and in the Certain Cure of Several Others; Particularly the Gravel, Asthmas,
Coughs, Hoarseness, and a Tough Morning Phlegm;* reprinted by Richard Jones, "Honey
and Healing," *Bee World* 78, no. 3 (1997): 146-149. Hill was an interesting per-
sonality: doctor, scientist, and prolific writer, having authored some 70 total volumes. The above book is filed at the IBRA library, U.K. A short biography of Hill
was also published: B. Hill, "Jack of All Trades: the Life of 'Sir' John Hill, M.D.,"
Practitioner 165 (1950): 634-638.

p. 9

2nd paragraph (editorial). A. Zumla and A. Lulat, "Honey: A Remedy
Rediscovered," *J. of the Royal Soc. of Medicine* 82 (1989): 384-385.

Antibacterial Properties of Honey

p.10

Osmolarity section. The high osmolarity of honey might be expected to
desiccate wound tissue, but the osmotic flow of fluid from the wound is offset by
an inward flow from underlying tissues. See Cheryl Dunford, "Using Honey As
a Dressing for Infected Skin Lesions," *NT Plus* 96, no. 14 (April 6, 2000): 7-9.

pH section. Although honey has a low pH, it is also weakly buffered, that
is, its pH can readily rise when exposed to alkaline materials. Other acids (e.g.,
hydrochloric, sulfuric) require considerable alkaline additions to effect a pH
change (i.e., they are strongly buffered).

p.11

(To become active...). A.I. Schepartz and M.H. Subers, "The Glucose Oxidase of Honey 1. Purification and some General Properties of the Enzyme," *Biochimica et Biophysica Acta* 85 (1964): 228-237. Cited in Peter Molan's 1992 *Bee World* review.

p.11

(Could man ...) The alert reader might ask why a company couldn't simply mix glucose and glucose oxidase, adjust the pH to 3 or 4 (using gluconic acid or a similar noncaustic, weakly buffered acid) and essentially duplicate the H_2O_2 release mechanism in honey. That seems possible, although the final product wouldn't have all the other medicinal components of honey; and, such a man-made product would probably cost at least ten times as much as honey because it would be patented. (Although some feel that bees have a decipherable language, bees have neither the time nor the temperament to go through the red tape involved in getting a patent, to say nothing of the potential hazards while standing in lines). There are some patented colloidal materials that can release H_2O_2 over a period of time, but they have not proven to be as effective as honey. See L.Y. Chung, et al. "A Study of Hydrogen Peroxide Generation by, and Antioxidant Activity of, Granuflex (DuoDERM) Hydrocolloid Granules and Some Other Hydrogel/Hydrocolloid Wound Management Materials," *British Journal of Dermatology* 129, no. 2 (1993): 145-153.

p.12

(Floral nectar components). Medicinal properties of various honeys will be elucidated in coming years. Progress in this area can be followed on www.honey.com.

(Flavonoids...). S. Bogdanov "Characterisation of Antibacterial Substances in Honey," *Lebensmittel Wissenschaft Technologie* 17, no. 2 (1984): 74-76; quoted by Patricia Wit, *Honey and Healing*, (London: IBRA, 2001).

Other Health Benefits

p. 13

Peter Molan, *Bee World* 82, *no. 1* (2001): 22-40; see Chapter 26. The four headings listed here are discussed with references in Molan's review.
S. Frankel et al., "Antioxidant Activity and Correlated Characteristics of 14 Unifloral Honeys," *J. of Apicultural Research* 37, no. 1 (1998): 27-31. Molan's review (above) states that honey scavenges free radicals to prevent them from harming tissue.

L.Y. Chung et al., *British J. of Dermatology* 129, no. 2: 145-153; and by B. Halliwell, "How to Characterize a Biological Antioxidant," *Free Radic Res Commun*

9: 1-32. The apparent paradox of a compound having both oxident properties (by producing H202) and antixoxidant properties was addressed in these articles.

Last sentence (Manuka honey). Peter Molan, personal communication.

Honey for Wounds

p. 14

Opening poem. Bodog Beck, *Honey and Health* (New York: Robert McBride, 1938).

1st anecdote (Bulgarian soldiers). T.M. Dobrovsky, "The Disinfecting and Healing Properties of Honey," *Bee Culture* (Dec. 1983): 648, 656, 658.

2nd anecdote (War invalid S.). N. Yoirish, *Curative Properties of Honey and Bee Venom* (San Francisco: New Glide Publications, 1977). Yoirish quotes a Ukrainian doctor, A. Budai.

p.15

3rd ancecdote (stomach incision). Alan R. Gaby, "Literature Review and Commentary," *Townsend Letter for Doctors* 143 (June 1995): 25.

4th anecdote (A severe case...). C. Dunford, R.A. Cooper and P.C. Molan, "Using Honey as a Dressing for Infected Skin Lesions," *Nurs Times* 96 (2000 NT Plus 14): 7-9.

p.16

(For treatment of burst abdominal wounds...). W. Phuapradit and N. Saropala, "Topical Application of Honey in Treatment of Abdominal Wound Disruption," *Australian and New Zealand Journal of Obstetrics and Gynecology* 32, no. 4 (1992): 381-384.

(In several other studies...). Peter Molan's 1999 review article in *Bee World* 80, no. 2, (1999): 80-92.

(A 1998 study reported...). A. Vardi et al., (1998) "Local Application of Honey for Treatment of Neonatal Postoperative Wound Infection," Acta Paediatr 87, no. 4 (1998): 429-432; cited by P. Molan, "Potential of Honey in the Treatment of Wounds and Burns," *Amer Journal Clinical Dermatology* 20 (2000): 13-19.

(In a 1994 study...) S. Harris "Honey for the Treatment of Superficial Wounds: a Case Report and Review," *Primary Intention Aust J Wound Manager* 2, no. 4 (1994): 18-23; cited by Molan in his 1999 and 2001 reviews, above.

(list of wounds). From Molan's 1999 *Bee World* Review, above. A few of Molan's references to this list are to anecdotes, but most are to scientific studies.

p.17

(Why honey is a superior wound dressing). See pages 27 and 28 of Molan's

2001 *Bee World* review 82, no. 1 (2001): 22-40.

(Using honey as a dressing) Peter Molan and Julie Betts, "Using Honey Dressings: the Practical Considerations," *Nursing Times* 96, no. 49 (Dec. 7, 2000): 36-37. This article outlines using honey dressings.

p.18

Last paragraph. C. Dunford et al., "The Use of Honey in Wound Management," *Nursing Standard* 15, no. 11 (Nov. 9, 2000): 63-68.

Last sentence. Thomas A. Mustoe, "Invited Critique [of Study of Honey and Wounds]," *Archives of Surgery* 135 (2000): 1417

Honey for Burns

p. 19

1st paragraph. T.M. Dobrvosky, "The Disinfecting and Healing Properties of Honey," *Bee Culture* (Dec. 1983): 648, 656, 658.

2nd paragraph. Robert Berthold, "Medicinal Use of Honey in Folk Medicine," *American Bee Journal* (Dec. 1997): 872-873.

(Three studies). 1. M. Subrahmanyam, "Topical Application of Honey in Treatment of Burns," *British Journal of Surgery* 78 (1991): 497-498; 2. M. Subrahmanyam, "Honey-impregnated Gauze Versus Polyurethane Film (OpSite) in the Treatment of Burns—a Prospective Randomised Study," *British Journal of Plastic Surgery* 46, no. 4 (1993): 322-323; 3. M. Subrahmanyam, "Honey-impregnated Gauze Versus Amniotic Membrane in the Treatment of Burns," *Burns* 20, no. 4 (1994): 331-333.

p.20

(Netherlands scientist quote). Theo Postmes, "The Treatment of Burns and Other Wounds with Honey," *Honey and healing* (Cardiff, UK: IBRA, 2001), pp. 42-47.

Honey for Stomach Problems

p.20

anecdotes, T.M. Dobrovsky, "The Disinfecting and Healing Properties of Honey," *Bee Culture* (Dec. 1983): 648, 656, 658.

p.21

anecdotes, N. Yoirish, *Curative Properties of Honey and Bee Venom* (San Francisco: New Glide Publications, 1977)

Science, 1st sentence. It is now accepted that at least 70% of stomach ulcers are caused by *H. pylori* (the remaining 30% are caused by aspirin and related medications). *H. pylori* was shown to be the culprit in stomach ulcers in the early

1980s by Australian scientist Barry marshall. Marshall's work flew in the face of conventional wisdom on ulcers—that ulcers were caused mainly stress and by spicy foods. It took time for Marshall's ideas to be accepted, but today ulcers are routinely treated with antibiotics. The story of Marshall's work is an intriguing one. There are several websites devoted exclusively to *H. pylori* and to Dr. Marshall: www.helicobacter.com, www. hpylori.com.au/, www. helico.com and others. See also Nancy Lynch, "Helicobacter and Ulcers: a Paradigm Revised," www.faseb.org/opar/pylori/pylori.html.

A related bacteria species, *Camplobacter pylori*, had been implicated in a number of disorders of the gastrointestinal tract before Marshall's work on *H. pylori*. Two California doctors give a good review of *C. pylori*: C. Dooley and H. Cohen, "The Clinical Significance of Camplobacter pylori," *Annals of Internal Medicine* 108 (1989): 70-79.

Science, 2nd sentence. A.I. Ali, "Inhibitory Effect of Natural Honey on *Helicobacter pylori*," *Tropical Gastroenterology* 12, no. 3 (1991): 139-143.

Science, 3rd sentence. A.I. Somai et al., "Susceptibility of *Helicobacter pylori* to the Antibacterial Activity of Manuka Honey," *Journal of the Royal Society of Medicine* 87, no. 1 (1994): 9-12.

2nd paragraph (Researchers at Hebrew…). The Hebrew University study was reported in the *National Examiner*, April 26, 1994, and reprinted in the May 1994 *Speedy Bee*, where I saw it. The reader can make his or her own judgment on the reliability of the source.

3rd paragraph (Science). O.A. Al-Swayeh and A.T.M. Ali, "Effect of Ablation of Capsaicin-Sensitive Neurons on Gastric Pprotection by Honey and Sucralfate," *HepataGastroenterology* 45, no. 19 (1998): 297-302; and A.T.M. Ali and O.A. Al-Swayeh, "The Role of Nitric Oxide in Gastric Protection by Honey," *Saudi Medical Journal* 11, no. 4 (1996): 275-279.

p.22

(There are numerous anecdotes…). N. Yoirish, *Curative Properties of Honey and Bee Venom* (San Francisco: New Glide Publications, 1977).

(In general, antibiotics give a dramatic…). "Drugs Counteract Irritable Bowel Syndrome," *Science News* v. 153 (Dec. 23, 30). The work was done by gastrotenerologist Mark Pimental and his colleagues at Cedars-Sinai Medical Center and the University of California, Los Angeles.

(In a test…). I.E. Haffejee and A. Moosa, "Honey in the Treatment of Infantile Gastroenteritis," *British Medical Journal* 290 (1985): 1866-1867.

Honey for Infants

p. 22

Opening paragraph. *Bee Culture* 114 (1986): 105. The consensus of those that have studied infant botulism in depth is that the threat has been greatly exaggerated. According to this report:

Dr. C. N. Huhtanen of the Eastern Utilization Laboratory in his recent address at the American Beekeeping Federation convention pointed out, "It's impossible to build a case associating infant botulism exclusively with honey." At least 80% of infant botulism cases have never had any contact with honey. In a Food and Drug Administration study of foods associated with infant feeding, eight samples of corn syrup out of a total of 40 were found to contain botulism spores. In the same test of 200 honey samples only two were found to contain spores.

In a study by Dr. Long of Pennsylvania, breast feeding was found to be associated with all infant botulism cases. Dr. Huhtanen said "It should be pointed out to pediatricians that breast feeding is a much greater risk factor in infant botulism than honey."

A recent review of botulism in Honey and healing (2001) IBRA (see Other Sources) reaches pretty much the same conclusion and lists 26 references on the subject.

Two good articles on honey and botulism are:

Wade Lawrence (D.V.M.), "Infant Botulism and its Relationship to Honey: a Review," *American Bee Journal* 126 (1986): 484-486; and Dr. Jill Snowden, "Infant Botulism," *Bee Culture* 120 (1992):2022.

p.23

3rd paragraph (1938 study). F.W. Schultz and E.M. Knott, "The Use of Honey as a Carbohydrate in Infant Feeding," *Journal of Pediatrics* 13 (Oct. 1938): 465-473.

Personal note: my three children were given one to two teaspoonfuls of honey in their bottles from age three months to 18 months. They slept through the night at every age and had regular, normal bowel movements. This was in the 1960s.

(Hemoglobin). N. Yoirish, *Curative Properties of Honey and Bee Venom* (San Francisco: New Glide Publications, 1977). Yoirish mentions this in his book.

Dr. Bodog Beck, *Honey and Health* (New York: Robert McBride, 1938) Beck cites two European studies that indicated honey increased blood hemoglobin. In one, 100 children were divided into two groups; half received honey (one to two tablespoons a day), half did not. After six weeks, the honey group showed a 12% increase in hemoglobin content of the blood. In a similar, but separate, Austrian study with 58 children, the half that received honey showed an 8.5% increase in hemoglobin.

p.24

Last paragraph (SIDS study). J.R. Kerr, et al., "An Association Between Sudden Infant Death Syndrome (SIDS) and "Helicobacter pylori Infection," *Archives of Diseases in Childhood* 83 (2000): 429-434. This study cites three other papers by C.P. Patterson et al. that indicated a link between SIDS and *H. pylori*; all three papers were published in *Gastroenterology*: "Is *Helicobacter pylori* the Missing Link for Sudden Infant Death Syndrome?" 112 (1997): A254; "Prevalence of *Helicobacter pylori* in Sudden Infant Death Syndrome," 114 (1998): G3688; "Confirmation of *Helicobacter pylori* by PCR in Sudden Infant Death Syndrome," 114 (1998): G3686.

It should be mentioned that the SIDS Alliance in an October 25, 2000, advisory stated that "alarming the public prematurely about any perceived relationship between *H. Pylori* and SIDS is unwarrented at this time." The SIDS Alliance suggested that the absence of *H. pylori* in seven of the eight control group members on the Kerr study cited above could have been due to some of the control group receiving antibiotics or being in a sterilized (hospital) environment. Certainly, more work needs to be done to prove or disprove a link between *H. pylori* and SIDS. For current information on SIDS, see www.sidsalliance.org or call the Alliance at (800) 221-7437.

p.24

(The honey industry…) Methods other than gamma irradiation to rid honey of botulism spores are being tried. *American Bee Journal* (Jan 2002): 47-49 (reporting on University of Georgia study cited by the Honey Board).

Data on whether SIDS deaths increased after honey was essentially banned for infants may be impossible to come by since statistics on SIDS deaths were only initiated in 1979, the same year reports of botulism from honey came out. In recent years, SIDS deaths have dropped significantly, due in large part to a Back to Sleep campaign (putting infants on their backs to sleep), but an estimated 6,000 SIDS deaths still occur each year.

Honey for the Eyes

p.24

Opening quote. Bodog Beck, *Honey and Healing* (New York: Robert McBride, 1938).

p.25

Anecdotes, 1st sentence (Aristotle quote). Aristotle, Historia Animalium v. IV, trans. by D. Thompson; In *The Works of Aristotle*, edited by J. Smith, W. Ross. (Oxford, UK: Oxford University, 1910).

(Lotus honey, India). M.R. Fotidar and S.N. Fotidar "Lotus Honey," *Indian Bee Journal* 7 (1945): 102.

(Mayan information and honey eyedrops). Patricia Vit, "Stingless Bee Honey and the Treatment of Cataracts," chapter in *Honey and healing* (Cardiff, UK: IBRA, 2001), 37-40.

2nd paragraph. N. Yoirish, *Curative Properties of Honey and Bee Venom* (San Francisco: New Glide Publications, 1977).

3rd paragraph (horse). *American Bee Journal* (July 1937): 350.

4th paragraph (Dr. Carey). Fred Malone, *Bees Don't Get Arthritis* (New York: E.P. Dutton, 1979), p. 49.

p.26

Science, 1st paragraph (102 patients). M.H. Emarah, "A Clinical Study of the Topical Use of Bee Honey in the Treatment of some Occular Diseases," *Bulletin of Islamic Medicine* 2, no. 5 (1982): 422-425. Cited by Peter Molan in his 1999 *Bee World* review; see Molan's Mountain.

2nd paragraph. Patricia Vit, "Stingless Bee Honey and the Treatment of Cataracts," chapter in *Honey and healing* (Cardiff, UK: IBRA, 2001), 37-40.

Honey for the Skin

p.26

The information from this chapter is from a 1998 Honey Board brochure, now out of print, and from their website: www.honey.com. The Honey Board offices are located at 390 Lashley St., Longmont, CO 80501, (303) 776-2337.

Honey for Other Maladies

p. 28

(Hangovers). p. 263. Several references are cited. Eva Crane, ed. *Honey* (London: Heinemann, 1975).

(Cramps). D.C. Jarvis, *Folk Medicine* (Holt, Rinehart and Winston: 1958; reprinted Fawcett Crest Books: 1970), p. 112. See also Eva Crane, ed., *Honey* (London: Heinemann, 1975).

(Liver problems). N. Yoirish, *Curative Properties of Honey and Bee Venom* (San Francisco: New Glide Publications, 1977).

p. 29

(Dental health). Honey Board news release, reprinted in *American Bee Journal* (May 2001). See also Eric Mussen, "Honey and Your Teeth," U.C. Apiaries (Sep./Oct. 2001); and Pelczar, Chan and Krieg, *Microbiology* (1986), pp. 681-682, cited by Mussen.

2nd paragraph (Dental health). October 2001 wire service report citing a recent study in the *Archives of Internal Medicine*.

last paragraph (Honey and cancer). Connie Krochmal, "Anti-tumor Activities of Hive Products," *American Bee Journal* (June 1994): 420.

(*H. pylori* and stomach cancer). Naomi Uemura et al., "*Helicobacter pylori* and the Development of Gastric Cancer," *New England Journal of Medicine* 345, no. 11 (2000): 784-789.

p.30
    1st paragraph (mice study). Ismail Hamzaolglu et al., "Protective Covering of Surgical Wounds with Honey Impedes Tumor Implantation," *Archives of Surgery* 135 (Dec. 2000): 1414-1417.
    (Dr. Tonia Young-Farok quote). *Honey Producer* 33, no. 1 (2001): 21.
    2nd paragraph (1979 study). J.A. McDonald, et al., "Cancer Mortality Among Beekeepers," *Journal of Occupational Medicine* 21, no. 12 (Dec. 1979): 811-813. Also J.F. Fraumeni and R. Hoover, "Bee Venom Thought to Increase Cancer: Immunosurveillance and Cancer," *Epidemiologic Observations* (National Cancer Institute Monograph) 47 (1977): 121-126. Cited in the 1979 study by McDonald et al.

p.31
    (Miscellaneous problems, contraceptives). Richard Jones, "Honey and Healing Through the Ages," *Honey and healing* (Cardiff, UK: IBRA, 2001).
    Last sentence, 3rd paragraph). Peter Molan, personal communication (2001).

Do Germs Cause All Ailments?

p.32
    2nd paragraph (bacteria and heart disease). "New Hope for Ailing Hearts," *Health Magazine* (May 1999); Ulysses Torassa, "Bacteria and Asthma: A New Breath of Life," *San Francisco Chronicle* (Jan. 22, 2001): Science section.

Honey: A Remedy for Antibiotic Resistance

p.33
    2nd paragraph (John O. Hunter) *Science News* v. 158 (Dec. 23, 30, 2000): 405.

Honey for Hospitals

p.34
    The problem of antibiotic resistance has been widely disseminated by the media in recent years. *Time, Newsweek* and other magazines have run feature stories on the subject, as have the television networks. There is no need to document the problem here, but two quotes from a 1997 article are illustrative: Dr. Lucy Tompkins of Stanford University Medical Center and chairwoman of a conference covering the subject stated 'The horse is really out of the barn. We have not been nearly vigorous enough in policy and process to implement the systems

needed to prevent wide-scale [antibiotic] overuse." Dr. Jon Rosenberg, medical epidemiologist with the Emerging Infections Program of the California Department of Health Services, put it this way: "We're scraping the bottom of the barrel. This [the diminishing effectiveness of vancomycin] is predictive of future increases in serious infection, unless measures are taken to prevent the spread of vancomycin resistance." Lisa Krieger, "Resistant Bacteria on Rise in Bay Hospitals," *San Francisco Examiner* (Sept. 14, 1997).

Honey: A Medicine Without a Profit

p. 36,37

(There are, in fact,…) See Molan's website at http://honey/bio.waikato.ac.nz for further information.

Tests are currently being conducted on a number of different U.S. honeys to determine their antibacterial potency. Results of this testing can be followed on the Honey Board website, at www.honey.com.

PART II: HONEY FOR ATHLETES

The Ultimate Sports Drink

p.38

2nd paragraph. The Gatorade sales figures came from the 2000 Annual report of Quaker Oats Company.

p.39

(Sports drinks or…) The sugar content of sports drinks (or carbohydrate content, because all sugars are carbohydrates, and the carbohydrates in sports drinks are sugars) is usually given in grams (g) per 8 fluid ounces (one serving). To convert grams per 8 fluid ounces to pounds per gallon, multiply by 0.035 (e.g., 14 g per 8 oz serving = 0.49 lbs per gallon).

3rd paragraph. The sugar information for Gatorade and Powerade was taken from their 2001 labels. It is possible that either or both of these drinks will change their mix of sugars in coming years. Check the label.

4th paragraph. Dried honey products are used in the bakery trade, mainly as a matter of convenience. Dried honey could also be used as a sports supplement. To produce dried honey, the roughly 16% moisture level in liquid honey is reduced to around 2% by a variety of drying methods, some of them patented. The cost of dried honey (per pound of sugars) is comparable to liquid honey, but the advantages of dried honey less storage space, easier handling, better storability makes it a *niche* product for honey producers. Dried honey is not seen in grocery stores because honey is purchased mainly for taste, but backpackers have used the product and some bakers make extensive use of dried honey. See Joan

Manes Olstrom, "Dried Honey," *American Bee Journal* (Sept. 1983): 656-659.

5th paragraph. Lloyd Percival, "Experience with Honey in Athletic Nutrition," *American Bee Journal* (Oct. 1955).

p.40

Studies reported by the National Honey Board. See the Honey Board website at www.nhb.org or www.honey.com.

PART III: THE JOY OF HONEY *LA JOIE DU MIEL*

Kinds of Honey

p. 44

1st paragraph (Saw palmetto). Herbs have become a billion dollar industry in recent years. Many are harvested in the wild, but many (echinacea, ginko biloba, St. John's wort and others) are now being grown commercially on herb farms. Honey from bees placed on such a farm would be very interesting, although how many herbs have nectar-producing flowers is unknown to me at this time; check the next edition of this book.

Superior and Gourmet Honeys

p.44

1st quote (3rd paragraph). Kim Flottum, inner cover of *Bee Culture* (Sept. 1998): p. 6.

p.45

2nd quote (French honey). Mark Winston, "La Maison du miel" *Bee Culture* (April 1997): 21-22.

p.47

Last paragraph. During the five years that I was a hands-on beekeeper, the only honey I harvested from my hives was orange honey. After orange bloom in mid-April, bees in California usually make only enough honey (from alfalfa, cotton and melons) to carry them through the winter. Beekeepers fortunate enough to have the locations can make sage honey in June and buckwheat honey in July. Beekeeping is somewhat like dryland farming, and with California's rainless summers, pickings are slim for bees from July until almonds bloom in February (other than nearby irrigated farmland, where the bees are endangered by pesticides).

During peak orange bloom, which lasts less than a week, it is amazing how much nectar bees can collect. Orange blossoms are prolific nectar producers in most years, and bees can quickly get a full load of nectar from one flower rather than having to visit over 100 flowers, as is often the case the rest of the year. I left the bee business because orange growers were allowed to spray toxic chemicals during bloom, and bee colonies could be severely weakened by these sprays. The year after I sold out, rules were implemented that outlawed spraying during heavy orange bloom (a two- to three- week period).

p.48

3rd paragraph (A.I. Root quote). From Root, A.I. *ABC and XYZ of Bee Culture* (Medina, OH: A.I. Root, 1877) reprinted by Frank Pellet, *American Honey Plants* (Hamilton, IL: Dadant & Sons, 1976). Mt. Hymettus, in Greece, produces honey that was praised by the Roman scholar Pliny (A.D. 23-79). Honey from Hymettus attained a mythical status up to Root's time, but one hears little about it today, at least in the U.S.; should you visit Greece, you might inquire about Hymettus and its legendary honey.

p.49

18 honeys. These are my selections; others might choose differently, but their lists (if they reside in the U.S.) of the top ten honeys would likely include at least eight of these 18.

Toxic Honeys

p.51

Last of 3rd paragraph (uncapped honey). D.R. Olszowy, "Of Bees, Rhododendrons and Honey," *American Bee Journal* 117, no. 8 (1981): 498-500.

See also, Connie Krochmal, "Poison Honeys," *American Bee Journal* (Aug. 1994): 549, 550; and Karsten Munstedt and Uwe Lang "Honey—Risks and Adverse Effects," *American Bee Journal* (May 1998): 355-356.

Storing Honey

p.53

3rd paragraph (honey stored at 32° for five weeks). G.H. Austin "Maintaining High Quality in Liquid and Recrystalized Honey," *Canadian Bee Journal* 61, no. 1 (1953): 10-12, 20-23.

A good general reference on the subject is Ann Harman's "Storing Honey," *Bee Culture* (Nov. 2000): 43-45.

Buying Honey

p. 53

Opening song. Eva Crane, *Honey* (London: Heinemann, 1975), p. 447.

Recipes

p.57

1st paragraph (barbecue sauce). Sioux Bee puts out two types of BBQ sauce: "Original Style" and "Cajun Style" (hot). Sioux Bee's sauce is not available in some areas. I usually gave my clients honey at Christmas time, but substituted BBQ sauce for some, and now that's all they want.

Mead and Honey Ale

p. 57

Opening poem. Dr. Bodog Beck, *Honey and Health* (New York: Robert McBride, 1938), p. 218. It is noteworthy that the salutation "Skol," used to drink to the health of people, is a Scandinavian word derived from "skull."

p.58

4th paragraph. Roger Morse, *Making Mead* (Cheshire, CT: Wicwas Press, 1980), p. 127.

p. 59

Pict heather ale legend. Bodog Beck, *Honey and Health* ibid.
Theatrum Botanicum. Bodog Beck, *Honey and Health* ibid.

Last paragraph (Sioux Honey Ale). Lance Nixon, "Sue Bee Brand Lends Its Familiar Name to Beer," *Sioux Falls Argus Leader;* reprinted in *Honey Producer Magazine* 33, no. 2 (July 2001): 34.

Other Bee Products

p.60

1st paragraph. Justin Schmidt and Stephen Buchman, "Other Products of the Hive," in Graham, Joe ed. *The Hive and the Honey Bee* (Hamilton, IL: Dadant & Sons). This 62-page chapter gives a thoughtful and thorough coverage of this entire subject.

(Propolis.) (study on the dental cavities in rats). Michel Hyu Koo et al., "Propolis Thwarts Cavities," *The Week* (Sept. 14, 2001): 18.

For those wanting to delve further into propolis, there are a number of good reviews and articles:

E.L. Ghisalberti, "Propolis: A Review," *Bee World* 60, no. 2 (1979): 59-84.
W.T. Greenaway and F.R. Whatley, "The Composition and Plant Origins of Propolis: a Report of Work at Oxford," *Bee World* 71 (1990): 122-129.

P. Cheng and G. Wong, (1996) "Honey Bee Propolis: Prospects in Medicine," *Bee World* 77, no. 1 (1996): 8-15.

M.C. Marcucci, "Propolis: Chemical Composition, Biological Properties and Therapeutic Activity," *Apidologie* 26 (1995): 83-99.

J. Iannuzzi, "Propolis: The Most Mysterious Hive Element," *American Bee Journal* (Aug. 1983): 573-575, (Sept. 1983): 631-633.

Karsten Munstedt and Marek Zygmunt, "Propolis—Current and Future Medical Uses," *American Bee Journal* (July 2001): 507-510.

M.S. Paima and O. Malaspina, "Propolis" *BeeBiz* (Jan. 1999): 17-21.

p.61

(Venom). Fred Malone, *Bees Don't Get Arthritis* (New York: E.P. Dutton, 1979). This book recounts many stories of arthritis sufferers being helped by bee stings. Malone traveled the U.S. to seek out first-hand information, and his book is an enjoyable read on the subject.

Dog study. J.A. Vick et al., "The Effect of Treatment with Whole Bee Venom on Daily Cage Activity and Plasma Cortisol Levels in Arthritic Dogs," *American Bee Journal* 115 (1975): 52, 53, 58; also *Inflammation* 1 (1975-76): 167-174.

Charles Mraz, *Health and the Honeybee* (1995). In his book, Mraz gives case histories on his successful bee-sting treatments for arthritis and multiple sclerosis. Mraz has more than 50 years experience, and offers how-to guidelines for using bee venom.

For more on bee venom therapy see: www.beesting.com. The Apitherapy Society of America, www.apitherapy.org, holds annual (or bi-annual) meetings. See also, www.apitherapy.com and the apitherapy links on the IBRA site: www.ibra.org.uk.

In 1997, Christopher Kim, M.D., published a comprehensive literature review in *Potentiating Health and the Crisis of the Immune System*, edited by Mizahi et al. Plenum Press, New York.

p.62

(Wax). For beeswax candles, contact A.I. Root Co., Box 706 Medina, OH 44258; (800) 289-7668, for an outlet near you.

(Bee brood). I've tried raw bee brood and found it to be tasty. It's a very white, pearly, attractive product, unlike the larvae of some other insects.

Epilogue

p.63

2nd paragraph. Federal Bank of San Francisco Economic Letter (Dec. 14, 2001)

p.64

(quote to science students). W. Grierson, "The Enforced Conservatism of Young Horticultural Scientists," *Hort. Science* 15, no. 3 (1980): 228-229.

Molan's Mountain

A number of sources were used for this book, but there would be no book without Peter Molan's groundbreaking reviews.

In 1953 a New Zealand beekeeper, Edmund Hillary (now Sir Edmund Hillary) was the first to climb Mt. Everest. In the 1990s, another New Zealander, Peter Molan, undertook the formidable task of synthesizing a myriad of disparate reports on the medicinal benefits of honey into a coherent whole that is greater than the sum of its parts. Molan showed the inter-relatedness of these reports, emphasizing the theme that honey has antimicrobial properties that are quite useful in treating a number of maladies. Molan then dissected just what gives honey these antimicrobial properties.

Individually, these reports would have languished on library shelves or been treated as anomalies. Combined by Molan, they represent an impressive mountain that cannot be ignored by the medical community. Molan's compilations are a remarkable piece of scholarship, and when the day comes that honey is an (or *the*) accepted treatment for a number of different ailments—and that day will surely come—much of the credit will go to Molan.

Molan published two 2-part reviews in *Bee World*, the award-winning publication of the International Bee Research Association (IBRA):

"The Antibacterial Activity of Honey" (1992)
1. "The Nature of the Antibacterial Activity," 73 (1992): 5-28.
2. "Variation in the Potency of the Antibacterial Activity," 73 (1992): 59-76.

"Why Honey is Effective As a Medicine" (1999 and 2001)
1. "Its Use in Modern Medicine," 80 (1999): 80-92.
2. "The Scientific Explanation of Its Effects," 82 (2001): 22-40.

These publications are available from the International Bee Research Association (IBRA), 18 North Road, Cardiff, CF10 3DY, U.K. (England). Phone: (+44) 222 372409.

In 1999, Molan published the review article "Potential of Honey in the Treatment of Wounds and Burns," *American J. of Clinical Dermatology* 2, no. 1 (1999): 13-19.

Molan also authored or coauthored a number of hands-on studies of the medicinal benefits of honey and works at the Honey Research Unit, Dept. of Biological Sciences, University of Waikato, Hamilton, New Zealand.

Following is a compilation of references cited by Molan in his review articles. Not all of them deal specifically with honey as a medicine, but most of those that do so represent controlled scientific studies published in reputable journals. Molan's references are listed here not so much so that a person can look them up (although that is not discouraged), but in the hopes that the sheer volume of references will convince the skeptic that maybe there is something to honey as a medicine.

The following references are cited by Peter Molan in his 2001 *Bee World* review: "Why Honey Is Effective as a Medicine. 2. The scientific explanation of its effects. *Bee World* 82, no. 1: 22-40.

1. ABBAS, T (1997) Royal treat. *Living in the Gulf;* pp. 50-51

2. ABUHARFEIL, N; AL-ORAN, R; ABO-SHEHADA, M (1999) The effect of bee honey on the proliferative activity of human B- and T-lymphocytes and the activity of phagocytes. *Food and Agricultureal Immunology* 11: 169-177.

3.AGNER, K (1963) Studies on myeloperoxidse activity. 1. Spectrophotometry of the MPO-H_2O_2 compound. *Acta Chemica Scandivaca* 17 (Suppl. 1): S332-S338.

4.AKHTAR, M S; KHAN, M S (1989) Glycemic responses to three different honeys given to normal and alloxan-diabetic rabbits. *Journal of the Pakistan Medical Assocation* 39(4): 107-113.

5. AL-SWAYEH, O A; ALI, A T M (1998) Susceptibility of *Helicobacter pylori* to the antibacterial activity of Manuka honey. *Journal of the Royal Society of Medicine* 87(1): 9-12.

6. AL-SWAYEH,O A A; ALI, A T M (1998) Effect of ablation of capsaicin-sensative neurons on gastric protection by honey and sucralfate. *Hepato-Gastronterology* 45(19): 297-302.

7. ALI, A T M (1995) Natural honey accelerates healing of indomethacin-induced antral ulcers in rats. *Saudi Medical Journal* 16(2): 161-166.

8. ALI, A T M M (1991) Prevention of ethanol-induced gastric lesions in rats by natural honey, and its possible mechanism of action. *Scandinavian Journal of Gastroenterology* 26: 281-288.

9. ALI, A T M M (1995) Natural honey exerts its protective effects against ethanol-induced gastric lesions in rats by preventing depletion of glandular nonprotein sulfhydryls. *Tropical Gastroenterology* 16 (1): 18-26.

10. ALI, A T M M; AL-HUMAYYD, M S; MADAN, B R (1990) Natural honey prevents indomethacin- and ethanol-induced gastric lesions in rats. *Saudi Medical Journal* 11(4): 275-279.

11. ALI, A T M M; AL-SWAHYEH, O A (1996) The role of nitric oixide in gastric protection by honey. *Saudi Medical Journal* 17: 301-306.

12.ALI, A T M M; AL-SWAHYEH, O A (1997) Natural honey prevents ethanol-induced increased vascular permeability changes in the rat stomach. *Journal of Ethnopharmacology* 55(3): 231-238.

13. ALI, A T M M; AL-SWAHYEH, O A: AL-HUMAYYD, M S: MUSTAFA, A A; AL-RASHED, R S; AL-TUWAIJIRI, A S (1997) Natural honey prevents ischemia-reperfusion-induced gastric mucosal lesions and increased vascular permeability in rats. *European Journal of Gastroenterology and Hepatology* 9 (11): 1101-1107.

14. ALI, A T M M; CHOWDHURY, M N H; AL-HUMAYYD, M S (1991) Inhibitory effect of natural honey on *Helicobacter pylori*. *Tropical Gastroenterology* 12 (3): 139-143.

15. ALLEN, K L; MOLAN, P C (1997) The sensitivity of mastitis-casuing bacteria to the antibacterial acitivity of honey. *New Zealand Journal of Agricultural Research* 40: 537-540.

16. ARISTOTLE ((350 B.C.) 1910 *Historia Animalium*. Oxford University; Oxford, UK.

17. ARMON, P J (1980) The use of honey in the treatment of infected wounds. *Tropical Doctor* 10:91.

18. BAUER, L; KOHLICH, A; HIRSCHWEHR, R; SIEMANN, U; EBNER, H; SCHEINER, O; KRAFT, D; EBNER, C (1996) Food allergy to honey; pollen or bee products Characterisation of allergenic proteins in honey by means of immunoblotting. *Journal of Allergy and Clinical Immunology* 97(1): 65-73.

19. BLEFIELD, W O; GOLINSKY, S; COMPTON, M D (1970) The use of insulin in open wound healing. *Veterinary Medicine: Small Animal Clinician* 65(5): 455-460.

20. BERGMAN, A; YANAI, J; WEIAA, J; BELL, D; DAVID, M P (1983) Acceleration of wound healing by topical application of honey. An animal model. *American Journal of Surgery* 145:374-376.

21. BLOMFIELD, R (1973) Honey for decubitus ulcers. *Journal of the American Medical Association* 224(6): 905.

22. BLOOMFIELD, E (1976) Old remedies. *Journal of the Royal College of General Pracitioners* 26: 576

23. BOSE, B (1982) Honey or sugar in treatment of infected wounds? *Lancet* i(April24): 963.

24. BRADY, N F; MOLAN, P C; HARFOOT, C G (1977) The sensitivity of dermatophytes to the antimicrobial activity of Manuka honey and other honey. *Pharmaceutical Sciences* 2: 1-3.

25. BRANIKI, F J (1981) Surgery in Western Kenya. *Annals of the Royal College of Surgeons of England* 63: 348-352.

26. BROOKS, F P (1985) The pathophysiology of peptic ulcer disease. *Digestive Diseases and Sciences* 30(11): 15S-25S.

27. BUCKNALL, T E (1984) Factors affecting healing. In T E Bucknall H Ellis (eds) *Wound healing for surgeons*. BailliEre Tindall; London, UK; pp 42-74.

28. BULMAN, M W (1955) Honey as a surgical dressing. *Middlesex Hospital Journal* 55: 188-189.

29. BURDON R H (1995) Superoxide and hydrogen peroxide in relation to mammalian cell proliferation. *Free Radical Biology and Medicine* 18 (4): 775-794.

30. BURLANDO, F (1978) Sullíazione terapeutica del miele nelle ustioni. *Minerva Dermatologica* 113: 699-706.

31. CAVANAGH, D; BEAZLEY, J; OSTAPOWICZ, F (1970) Radical operation for carcinoma of the vulva. A new approach to wound healing. *Journal of Obstetrics and Gynecology of the British Commonwealth* 77(11): 1037-1040.

32. CHANT, A (1999) The biomechanics of leg ulceration. *Annals of the Royal College of Surgeons of England* 81: 80-85.

33. CHIRIFE, J; HERSZAGE, L; JOSEPH, A; KOHN, E S (1983) *In vitro* study of bacterial growth inhibition in concentrated sugar solutions; microbiological basis for the use of sugar in treating infected wounds. *Antimicrobial Agents and Chemotherapy* 23(5): 766-773.

34. CHUNG, L Y; SCHMIDT, R J; ANDREWS, A M; TURNER, T D (1993) A study of hydrogen peroxide generation by, and antioxidant activity of, Granuflex (DuoDERM) hydrocolloid granules and some other hydrogel/hydrocolloid wound management materials. *British Journal of Dermatology* 129 (2): 145-153.

35. CHURCH, J (1954) Honey as a source of the anti-stiffness factor. *Federation Proceedings of the American Physiology Society* 13(1): 26.

36. COCHRANE, C G (1991) Cellular injury by oxidants. *American Journal of Medicine* 91(Suppl. 3c): 23S30S.

37. COOPER, R A; MOLAN, PC (1999) The use of honey as an antiseptic in managing *Pseudomonas* infection. *Journal off Wound Care* 8(4): 161-164.

38. COOPER, R A; MOLAN, P C; HARDING, K G (1999) Antibacterial activity of honey against strains of *Staphylococcus aureus* from infected wounds. *Journal of the Royal Society of Medicine* 92: 283-285.

39. CROSS, C E; HALLIWELL, B; BORISH, E T; PRYOR, W A; AMES, B N; SAUL, R L; MCCORD, J M; HARMAN, D (1987) Oxygen radicals and human disease. *Annals of Internal Medicine* 107: 526545.

40. CURDA, L; PLOCKOV, M (1995) Impedance measurement of growth of lactic acid bacteria in dairy cultures with honey addition. *International Dairy Journal* 5: 727-733.

41. CZECH, M P; LAWRENCE Jr, J C; LYNN, W S (1974) Evidence for the involvement of sulphydryl oxidation in the regulation of fat cell hexose transport by insulin. *Proceedings of the National Academy of Sciences of the United States of America* 71(10): 4173-4177.

42. DAILEY, L A; IMMING, P (1999) 12 Lipoxygenase: classification, possible therapeutic benefits from inhibition and inhibitors. *Current Medical Chemistry* 6(5): 389-398.

43. DAVIS, C; ARNOLD, K (1974) Role of meningococcal endotoxin in meningococcal purpura. *Journal of Experimental Medicine* 140: 159-171.

44. DEFORGE, L E; FANTONE, J C; KENNEY, J S; REMICK, D G (1992) Oxygen radical scavengers selectively inhibit interleukin B production in human whole blood. *Journal of Clinical Investigation* 90: 2123-2129.

45. DOOLEY, C P; COHEN, H (1989) The clinical significance of *Campylobacter pylori*. *Annals of Internal Medicine* 108: 70-79.

46. DUMRONGLERT, E (1983) A follow-up study of chronic wound healing dressing with pure natural honey. *Journal of the National Research Council of Thailand* 15(2): 39-66.

47. DUNFORD, C; COOPER, R A; MOLAN, P C (2000) Using honey as a dressing for infected skin lesions. *Nursing Times* 96 (NTPLUS 14): 79.

48. DUNFORD, C; COOPER, R A; WHITE, R J; MOLAN, P C (2000) The use of honey in wound management. *Nursing Standard* 15(11): 63-68.

49. EFEM, S E E (1988) Clinical observations on the wound healing properties of honey. *British Journal of Surgery* 75: 679-681.

50. EFEM, S. E E (1993) Recent advances in the management of Fournier's gangrene: preliminary observations. *Surgery* 113(2): 200-204.

51. EFEM, S E E; Udoh, K T; Iwara,C I (1992) The antimicrobial spectrum of honey and its clinical significance. *Infection* 20(4): 227-229.

52. EL-BANBY, M; KANDIL, A; ABOU-SEHLY, G; EL-SHERIF, M E; ABDEL-WAHED, K. Healing effect of floral honey and honey from sugar-fed bees on surgical wounds (animal model). In IBRA (eds) 4th International Conference on Apikulture in Tropical Climates, 1989, Cairo. *International Bee Research Association*; Cardiff, UK.

53. EL-SUKHON, S N; ABU-HARFEIL, N; SALLAL, A K (1994) Effect of honey on bacterial growth and spore germination. *Journal of Food Protection* 57(10): 918-920.

54. EMARAH, M H (1982) A clinical study of the topical use of bee honey in the treatment of some occular diseases. *Bulletin of Islamic Medicine* 2(5): 422-425.

55. FAROUK, A; HASSAN, T; KASHIF, H; KHALID, S A; MUTAWALI, I; WADI, M (1988) Studies on Sudanese bee honey: laboratory and clinical evaluation. *International Journal of Crude Drug Research* 26(3): 161-168.

56. FLOHE, L; BECKMANN, R; GIERTZ, H; LOSCHEN, G (1985) Oxygen-centred free radicals as mediators of inflammation, In H Sies (ed) *Oxidative Stress*. Academic Press; London, UK; pp 403-435.

57. FLORIS, I; PROTA, R (1989) Sul miele amaro di Sardegna. *Apicoltore Moderno* 80(2): 55-67.

58. FORDTRAN, J S (1975) Stimulation of active and passive sodium absorption by sugars in the human jejunum. *Journal of Clinical Investigation* 55: 728-737.

59. FOTIDAR, M R; FOTIDAR, S N (1945) Lotus honey. *Indian Bee Journal* 7: 102.

60. FRANKEL, S; ROBINSON, G E; BERENBAUM, M R (1998) Antioxidant capacity and correlated characteristics of 14 unifloral honeys. *Journal of Apicultural Research* 37(1): 27-31.

61. GRIMBLE, G F (1994) Nutritional antioxidants and the modulation of inflammation: theory and practice. *New Horizons* 2(2): 175-185.

62. GUNTHER, R T (1934 (Reprinted 1959)) *The Greek herbal of Dioscorides.* Hafner; New York; 701 pp.

63. GUPTA, S K; SINGH, H; VARSHNEY A C; PRAKASH, P (1992) Therapeutic efficacy of honey in infected wounds in buffaloes. *Indian Journal of Animal Sciences* 62(6): 521-523.

64. HAFFEJEE, I E; MOOSA, A (1985) Honey in the treatment of infantile gastroenteritis. *British Medical Journal* 290: 1866-1867.

65. HALLIWELL, B; CROSS, C E (1994) Oxygen-derived species: Their relation to human disease and environmental stress. *Environmental Health Perspectives* 102 Suppl 10: 5-12.

66. HARRIS, S (1994) Honey for the treatment of superficial wounds: a case report and review. *Primary Intention* 2(4): 18-23.

67. HASPOLAT, K; BYUKBAS, S; ENGEL, H (1990) Balin in vicro antibakteriyel ve antifungal etkisi. *Turk Hijiyen ve Deneysel Byoloji Dergisisi* 47(2): 211-216.

68. HAURY B; RODEHEAVER, G; VENSKO, J; EDGERTON, M T; EDLICH, R F (1978) Debridement: an essential component of traumatic wound care. *American Journal of Surgery* 135: 238-242.

69. HAYDAK, M H (1955) The nutritional value of honey. *American Bee Journal* 95: 185-191.

70. HEJASE, M J; E., S J; BIHRLE, R; COOGAN, C L (1996) Genital Fournier's gangrene: experience with 38 patients. *Urology* 47(5): 734-739.

71. HELBLING, A; PETER, C; BERCHTOLD, E; BOGDANOV, S; MOLLER, U (1992) Allergy to honey: relation to pollen and honeybee allergy. *Allergy* 47(1): 41-49.

72. HELM, B A; GUNN, J M (1986) The effect of insulinomimetic agents on protein degradation in H35 hepatoma cells, *Molecular and Cellular Biochemistry* 71(2): 159-166.

73. HUNT, T K; TWOMEY, P; ZEDERFELDT, B; DUNPHY, J E (1967) Respiratory gas tensions and pH in healing wounds. *American Journal of Surgery* 114: 302-307.

74. HUTTON, D J (1966) Treatment of pressure sores. *Nursing Times* 62(46): 1533-1534.

75. HYSLOP, P A; HINSHAW, D B; SCRAUFSTATTER, I U; COCHRANE, C G; KUNZ, S; VOSBECK, K (1995) Hydrogen peroxide as a potent bacteriostatic antibiotic: implications for host defense. *Free Radical Biology and Medicine* 19(1): 317.

76. JONES, K P; BLAIR, S; TONKS, A; PRICE, A; COOPER, R (2000) Honey and the stimulation of inflammatory cytokine release from a monocytic cell line. *First World Wound Healing Congress;* Melbourne, Australia.

77. KANDIL, A; EL-BANBY M ABDEL-WAHED, K; ABOU-SEHLY, G; EZZAT, N (1987) Healing effect of true floral and false nonfloral honey on medical wounds. *Journal of Drug Research* (Cairo) 17(12): 71-75.

78. KATSILAMBROS, N I; PHILIPPIDES, P; TOULIATOU, A; GEORGAKOPOULOS, K; KOFOTZOULI. L; FRANGAKI, D; SISKOUDIS, P; MARANGOS, M; SFIKAKIS, P (1988) Metabolic effects of honey (alone or combined with other foods) in Type 11 diabetics. *Acto Diabetologica Latina* 25: 197-203.

79. KAUFMAN, T; EICHENLAUB, E H; ANGEL, M F; LEVIN, M; FUTRELL, I W (1985) Topical acidification promotes healing of experimental deep partial thickness skin burns: a randomised double-blind preliminary study. *Burns* 12: 84-90.

80. KAUFMAN, T; LEVIN, M; HURWITZ, D J (1984) The effect of topical hyperalimentation on wound healing rate and granulation tissue formation of experimental deep second degree burns in guinea-pigs. *Burns* 10(4): 252-256.

81. KEAST-BUTLER, J (1980) Honey for necrotic malignant breast ulcers. *Lancet ii* (October 11): 809.

82. KIISTALA, R; HANNUKSELA, M; MAKINEN-KILJUNEN, S; NIINIMAKI, A; HAAHTELA, T (1995) Honey allergy is rare in patients sensitive to pollens. *Allergy* 50: 844-847.

83. KLEBANOFF, S J (1980) Myeloperoxidase-mediated cytotoxic systems. In A J Sbarra; R R Strauss (eds) The reticuloendothelial system. A comprehensive treatise. Volume 2. *Biochemistry and Metabolism.* Plenum Press; New York; pp 270-308.

84. KOSHIO, O; AKANUMA, Y; KASUGA, M (1988) Hydrogen peroxide stimulates tyrosine phosphorylation of the insulin receptor and its tyrosine kinase activity in intact cells. *Biochemical Journal* 250: 95-101.

85. KUMAR, A; SHARMA, V K; SINGH, H P; PRAKASH, P; SINGH, S P (1993) Efficacy of some indigenous drugs in tissue repair in buffaloes. *Indian Veterinary Journal* 70(1): 42-44.

86. LEVEEN, H H; FALK, G; BOREK, B; DIAZ, C; LYNFIELD, Y; WYNKOOR B I; MABUNDA, G A; RUBRICUS, J L; CHRISTOUDIAS, G C (1973) Chemical acidification of wounds. An adjuvant to healing and the unfavourable action of alkalinity and ammonia. *Annals of Surgery* 178(6): 745-753.

87. LINEAWEAVER, W; MCMORRIS, S; SOUCY D; HOWARD, R (1985) Cellular and bacterial toxicities of topical antimicrobials. *Plastic and Reconstructive Surgery* 75(3); 394-396.

88. LINNETT P (1996) Honey for equine diarrhea. *Control and Therapy:* 906.

89. LOPEZ. J E; MENA, B (1968) Local insulin for diabetic gangrene. *Lancet* i: 1199.

90. MCGOVERN, D P B; ABBAS, S Z; VIVIAN, G; DALTON, H R (1999) Manuka honey against *Helicobacter pylori. Journal of the Royal Society of Medicine* 92: 439.

91. MCINERNEY, R J F (1990) Honey, remedy rediscovered. *Journal of the Royal Society of Medicine* 83: 127.

92. MOLAN, P C (1992) The antibacterial activity of honey. 1. The nature of the antibacterial activity. *Bee World* 73(1): 528.

93. MOLAN, P C (1992) The antibacterial activity of honey. 2. Variation in the potency of the antibacterial activity. *Bee World* 73(2): 59-76.

94. MOLAN, P C (1998) A brief review of honey as a clinical dressing. *Primary Intention* 6(4): 148-158.

95. MOLAN P C (1999) Selection of honey for use as a wound dressing. *Primary Intention* (in press).

96. MOLAN, P C (1999) Why honey is effective as a medicine. 1. Its use in modern medicine. *Bee World* 80(2): 80-92.

97. MOLAN, P C; Allen, K L (1996) The effect of gamma irradiation on the antibacterial activity of honey. *Journal of Pharmacy and Pharmacology* 48: 1206-1209.

98. MOSSEL, D A A (1980) Honey for necrotic breast ulcers. *Lancet ii* (November 15): 1091.

99. MURPHY, G; REYNOLDS, J J; BRETZ, U; BAGGIOLINI, M (1982) Partial purification of collagenase and gelatinase from human polymorphonuclear leukocytes. *Biochemical Journal* 203: 209-221.

100. MURRELL, G A C; FRANCIS, M J O; BROMLEY, L (1990) Modulation of fibroblast proliferation by oxygen-free radicals. *Biochemical Journal* 265: 659-665.

101. NDAYISABA,G; BAZIRA, L; HABONIMANA, E; MUTEGANYA, D (1993) Clinical and bacteriological results in wounds treated with honey. *Journal of Orthopedic Surgery* 7(2): 202-204.

102. NIINIKOSKI, J; KIVISAARI, J; VILJANTO, J (1977) Local hyperalimentation of experimental granulation tissue. *Acto Chiropida Scandinavica* 143: 201-206.

103. NYCHAS, G J; DILLON, V M; BOARD. R G (1988) Glucose, the key substrate in the microbiological changes in meat and certain meat products. *Biotechnology and Applied Biochemistry* 10: 203

104. OBI, C L; UGOJI, E O; EDUN, S A; LAWAL, S F; ANYIWO, C E (1994) The antibacterial effect of honey on diarrhea-causing bacterial agents isolated in Lagos, Nigeria. *African Journal of Medical Sciences* 23: 257-260.

105. ORYAN, A; ZAKER, S R (1998) Effects of topical application of honey on cutaneous wound healing in rabbits. *Journal of Veterinary Medicine Series A* 45(3): 181-188.

106. OSSANNA, P J; TEST, S T; MATHESON, N R; REGIANI, S; WEISS, S J (1986) Oxidative regulation of neutrophil elastase-alpha-1-proteinase inhibitor interactions. *Journal of Clinical Investigation* 77: 1939-1951.

107. PEPPIN, G J; WEISS, S J (1986) Activation of the endogenous metalloproteinase, gelatinase, by triggered human neutrophils. *Proceedings of the National Academy of Sciences of the United States of America* 83: 4322-4326.

108. PHUAPRADIT, W; SAROPALA, N (1992) Topical application of honey in treatment of abdominal wound disruption. *Australian and New Zealand Journal of Obstetrics and Gynecology* 32(4): 381-384

109. PIERRE, E J; BARROW, R E; HAWKINS, H K; NGUYEN, T T; SAKURAI, Y; DESAI, M; WOLFE, R R; HERNDON, D N (1998) Effects of insulin on wound healing. *Journal of Trauma, Injury, Infection and Critical Care* 44 (2): 342-345.

110. POSTMES, T; BOGAARD, A E VAN DEN; HAZEN, M (1993) Honey for wounds, ulcers, and skin graft preservation. *Lancet* 341(8847): 756-757.

111. POSTMES, T; BOGAARD, A E VAN DEN; HAZEN, M (1995) The sterilization of honey with cobalt 60 gamma radiation: a study of honey spiked with *Clostridium botulinum* and *Bacillus subtilis. Experentia* (Basel) 51: 986-989.

112. POSTMES, T; VANDEPUTTE, J (1999) Recombinant growth factors or honey? *Burns* 25(7): 676-678.

113. POSTMES, T J; BOSCH, M M C; DUTRIEUX, R; BAARE, J VAN; HOEKSTRA, M J (1997) Speeding up the healing of burns with honey. An experimental study with histological assessment of wound biopsies. In A Mizrahi; Y Lensky (eds) *Bee products: properties, applications and apitherapy.* Plenum Press; New York; pp 27-37.

114. PRUITT, K M; REITER, B (1985) Biochemistry of peroxidase system: antimicrobial effects. In K M Pruitt; J O Tenovuo (eds) *The lactoperoxidose system chemistry and biological significance.* Marcel Dekker; New York; pp 144-178.

115. ROOS, D (1991) The respiratory burst of phagocytic leucocytes. *Drug Investigation* 3(suppl. 2): 49-53.

116. ROTH, LA; KWAN, S; SPORNS, P (1986) Use of a disc-assay system to detect oxytetracycline residues in honey. *Journal of Food Protection* 49(6): 436-441.

117. RYAN, G B; MAJNO, G (1977) *Inflammation.* Upjohn; Kalamazoo, Michigan, USA; 80 pp.

118. SAISSY, J M; GUIGNARD, B; PATS, B; GUIAVARCH, M; ROUVIER, B (1995) Pulmonary edema after hydrogen peroxide irrigation of a war wound. *Intensive Care Medicine* 21(3): 287-288.

119. SALAHUDEEN, A K; CLARK, E C; NATH, K A (1991) Hydrogen peroxide-induced renal injury. A protective role for pyruvate in vitro and in vivo. *Journal of Clinical Investigation* 88(6): 1886-1893.

120. SAMANTA, A; BURDEN, A C; JONES, G R (1985) Plasma glucose responses to glucose, sucrose, and honey in patients with diabetes mellitus: and analysis of glycemic and peak incremental indices. *Diabetic Medicine* 2(5): 371-373.

121. SCHRECK, R; RIEBER, P; BAEUERLE, P A (1991) Reactive oxygen intermediates as apparently widely used messengers in the activation of the NF-kB transcription factor and HIV-1. *EMBO Journal* 10(8): 2247-2258.

122. SHEIKH, D; SHAMS-UZ-ZAMAN; NAQVI, S B; SHEIKH, M R; ALI, G (1995) Studies on the antimicrobial activity of honey. *Pakistan Journal of Pharmaceutical Sciences* 8(1): 51-62.

123. SILVER, I A (1980) The physiology of wound healing. In T K Hunt (ed) *Wound healing and wound infection: theory and surgical practice.* Appleton-Century-Crofts; New York; pp 1128.

124. SILVETTI, A N (1981) An effective method of treating long-enduring wounds and ulcers by topical applications of solutions of nutrients. *Journal of Dermatolology, Surgery and Oncology* 7(6): 501-508.

125. SIMON, R H; SCOGGIN, C H; PATTERSON, D (1981) Hydrogen peroxide causes the fatal injury to human fibroblasts exposed to oxygen radicals. *Journal of Biological Chemistry* 256(14): 7181-7186.

126. SINCLAIR, R D; RYAN, T J (1994) Proteolytic enzymes in wound healing: the role of enzymatic debridement. *Australasian Journal of Dermatology* 35: 35-41.

127. SOMERFIELD, S D (1991) Honey and healing. *Journal of the Royal Society of Medicine* 84(3): 179.

128. SUBRAHMANYAM, M (1991) Topical application of honey in treatment of burns. *British Journal of Surgery* 78(4): 497-498.

129. SUBRAHMANYAM, M (1993) Honey impregnated gauze versus polyurethane film (OpSite(r)) in the treatment of burnsa prospective randomised study. *British Journal of Plastic Surgery* 46(4): 322-323.

130. SUBRAHMANYAM, M (1994) Honey-impregnated gauze versus amniotic membrane in the treatment of burns. *Burns* 20(4): 331-333.

131. SUBRAHMANYAM, M (1996) Honey dressing versus boiled potato peel in the treatment of burns: a prospective randomized study. *Burns* 22(6): 491-493.

132. SUBRAHMANYAM, M (1998) A prospective randomised clinical and histological study of superficial burn wound healing with honey and silver sulfadiazine. *Burns* 24(2): 157-161.

133. SUGUNA, L; CHANDRAKASAN, G; RAMAMOORTHY, U; THOMAS JOSEPH, K (1993) Influence of honey on biochemical and biophysical parameters of wounds in rats. *Journal of Clinical Biochemistry and Nutrition* 14: 91-99.

134. SUGUNA, L; CHANDRAKASAN, G; THOMAS JOSEPH, K (1992) Influence of honey on collagen metabolism during wound healing in rats. *Journal of Clinical Biochemistry and Nutrition* 13: 712.

135. SWAIM, S F (1980) *Surgery of traumatized skin: management and reconstruction in the dog and cat.* W B Saunders Co.; Philadelphia, USA; 120-122 pp.

136. TANAKA, H; HANUMADASS, M; MATSUDA, H; SHIMAZAKI, S; WALTER, R J; MATSUDA, T (1995) Hemodynamic effects of delayed initiation of antioxidant therapy (beginning two hours after burn) in extensive third-degree burns. *Journal of Burn Care and Rehabilitation* 16(6): 610-615.

137. TATNALL, F M; LEIGH, I M; GIBSON, J R (1991) Assay of antiseptic agents in cell culture: conditions affecting cytotoxicity. *Journal of Hospital Infection* 17(4): 287-296.

138. TONNESEN, M G; WORTHEN, G S; JOHNSTON, R B Jr. (1988) Neucrophil emigration, activation and tissue damage. In R A F Clark; P M Henson (eds) *The molecular and cellular biology of wound repair.* Plenum Press; New York, London; pp 149-183.

139. TUR, E; BOLTON, L; CONSTANTINE, B E (1995) Topical hydrogen peroxide treatment of ischemic ulcers in the guinea pig: Blood recruitment in multiple skin sites. *Journal of the American Academy of Dermatology* 3 3(2 Pt 1): 217-221.

140. TURNER. F J (1983) *Hydrogen peroxide and other oxidant disinfectants.* Lea & Febiger: Philadelphia. USA; 240-250 pp.

141. VARDI, A; BARZILAY, Z; LINDER, N; COHEN, H A; PARET, G; BARZILAI, A (1998) Local application of honey for treatment of neonatal postoperative wound infection. *Acto Poediatrica* 87(4): 429-432.

142. VILJANTO, J; RAEKALLIO, J (1976) Local hyperalimentation of open wounds. *British Journal of Surgery* 63: 427-430.

143. WADI, M; AL-AMIN, H; FAROUQ, A; KASHEF, H; KHALED, S A (1987) Sudanese bee honey in the treatment of suppurating wounds. *Arab Medico* 3: 16-18.

144. WAHDAN, H A L (1998) Causes of the antimicrobial activity in honey. *Infection* 36(1): 30-35.

145. WAKHLE, D M; DESAI, D B (1991) Estimation of antibacterial activity of some Indian honeys. *Indian Bee Journal* 53(14): 80-90.

146. WEBER. H (1937) *Honig zur Behandlung vereiterter Wunden. Therapie der Gegenwart* 78: 547.

147. WEHEIDA, S M; NAGUBIB, H H; EL-BANNA, H M; MARZOUK, S (1991) Comparing the effects of two dressing techniques on healing of low-grade pressure ulcers. Journal of the Medical Research Institute. Alexandria University 12(2): 259-278.

148. WEISS. S J; PEPPIN, G; ORTIZ, X; RAGSDALE, C; TEST, S T (1985) Oxidative autoactivation of latent collagenase by human neutrophils. *Science* 227: 747-749.

149. WHITE, J W (1975) Composition of honey. In E Crane (ed) *Honey: a comprehensive survey.* Heinemann; London, UK; pp. 157-206.

150. WILLIX, O J; MOLAN, P C; HARFOOT, C J (1992) A comparison of the sensitivity of wound-infecting species of bacteria to the antibacterial activity of Manuka honey and other honey. *Journal of Applied Bacteriology* 73: 388-394.

151. WINTER. G D (1962) Formation of the scab and the rate of epithelialization of superficial wounds in the skin of the young domestic pig. *Nature* (London) 193(4812): 293-294.

152. WOOD. B; RADEMAKER, M; MOLAN, P C (1997) Manuka honey, a low-cost, leg ulcer dressing. *New Zealand Medical Journal* 110: 107.

153. WORLD HEALTH ORGANISATION (1976) Treatment and prevention of dehydration in diarrhoeal diseases. *WHO*: 31 pp.

154. YANG, K L (1944) The use of honey in the treatment of chilblains, nonspecific ulcers, and small wounds. *Chinese Medical Journal* 62: 55-60.

155. ZAIB (1934) Der Honig in auBerlicher Anwendung. *Munchener Medizinische Wochenschrift* (49): 1891-1893.

The following references are cited by Peter Molan in his 1999 *Bee World* review that were not cited in his 2001 review. From Molan, P. (1999) "Why Honey Is Effective as a Medicine--Part 1 Its Use in Modern Medicine," *Bee World* 80, no. 2 (2001): 8-92.

Adsunkanmi, K; Oyelami, O.A. "The Pattern and Outcome of Burn Injuries at Wesley Guild Hospital, Ilesha, Nigeria: a Review of 156 cases." *J. of Tropical Medicine and Hygiene* 97, no.2 (1994): 108-112.

American Bee Journal. "Hospitals Using Honey as a Fast New Antibiotic." *American Bee Journal* 122, no. 4 (1982): 247.

Ankra-Badu, G.A. "Sickle Cell Leg Ulcers in Ghana." *East African Medical J.* 69, no. 7 (1992): 366-369.

Beck, B.F., D. Smedley. *Honey and Your Health*, 2nd Edition. New York: McBride, 1944.

Celsus (c. 25 A.D.). *De Medicina*. London: Heinemann.

Condon, R.E. "Curious Interaction of Bugs and Bees." *Surgery* 113, no. 2 (1993): 234-235.

Dany-Mazequ, MPG. "Honig auf die Wumde." *Krankenplege* 46, no. 1 (1992): 6-10.

Descotte, B. "De la ruche a l'hospital ou l'utilisation du miel dans l'unite de soins." *L'Abeille de France et l'Apiculture* 754 (1990): 459-460

Forrest, R.D. "Early History of Wound Treatment." *J. of the Royal Society of Medicine* 75 (1982): 198-205.

Green, A.E. "Wound Healing Properties of Honey." *British J. of Surgery* 75, no. 12 (1998): 1278

Greenwood, D. "Sixty Years on: Antimicrobial Drug Resistance Comes of Age." *Lancet* 346 (Supplement 1) (1995): s1

Khotkina, M.L. "Honey as Part of Therapy for Patients with Stomach Ulcers."

Collection of papers from the Irkutsk State Medical Institute. 1995: pp. 252-262. Lucke, H. "Wundbehandlung mit Honig und Lebertran." *Deutsche Medizinishe Wochenschrift* 61, no. 41 (1935): 1638-1640.

Menshikov, F.K., S.I. Fiedman. "Curing Stomach Ulcers with Honey." *Sovetskaya Meditsina* 10 (1949): 13-14.

Mladenov, S. Present problems of apitherapy, International Symposium on Apitherapy, 1974. Madrid, Bucharest, Romania: Apimondia Publishing House.

Mossel, D.A.A. "Honey for Necrotic Breast Ulcers." *Lancet ii* (Nov. 15, 1980: 1091.

Phillips, C.E. "Honey for Burns." Gleanings in *Bee Culture* 61 1993:84.

Popescu, P.P., E. Palos, F. Popescu. "Studiul eficacitati terapiei biologice complexe cu produse apicole in unele afectiuni oculare localizate palpebral si conjunctival in raport cu modificarile clinico-functionale." Revista de Chirugie Oncologie Radiologie ORL. *Oftalmologie Stomatologie Seria Oftalmologei* 29, no. 1 (1985): 53-61.

Salem, S.N. "Honey Regimen in Gastrointestinal Disorders." *Bulletin of Islamic Medicine* 1 (1981): 358-362.

Sarma, M.C. "Honey in the Treatment of Bacterial Corneal Ulcers." personal communication cited in Efem, S.E.E.: K. Udah, C. Iwara. "The Antimicrobial Spectrum of Honey and its Clinical Significance." *Infection* 20, no. 4 (1992): 227-229.

South African Medical Journal. Honey: Sweet and Dangerous or Panacea." *South African Medical Journal* 56 (1974): 2300.

Seymour, F.I., K.S. West. "Honey—It's Role in Medicine." *Medical Times* 79 (1951): 104-107.

Slobodianiuk, A.A., M. Slobodianiuk. Complex treatment of gastritis patients with high stomach secretion in combination with (and without) a 15-20% solution of honey. Ufa: Bashkir. Khniz. (1969) izd-vo.
Tovey, F.I. "Honey and Healing." *J. of the Royal Society of Medicine* 84, no. 7 (1991): 447.

The following references are cited by Peter Molan in his 1992 *Bee World* review that were not cited in his 1999 or 2001 reviews. *Bee World* 73, no. 1: 5-28, 73, no.2: 59-76.

1. ADCOCK, D (1962) The effect of catalase on the inhibine and peroxide values of various honeys. *Journal of Apicultural Research* 1: 38-40.

2. AGOSTINO BARBARO, A d'; ROSA, C La; ZANELLI, C (1961) Attivita antibatterica di mieli Siciliani. *Quaderni della Nutrizione* 21(1/2): 30-44.

3. ALLEN, K L; MOLAN, P C; REID, G M (1991) A survey of the antibacterial activity of some New Zealand honeys. *Journal of Pharmacy and Pharmacology* 43(12): 817-822.

4. AMOR, D M (1978) Composition, properties and uses of honey a literature survey. The British Food Manufacturing Industries Research Association; Leatherhead, UK; *Scientific and Technical Surveys* No.108; 84 pp (confidential).

5. BAIRD-PARKER, A C; HOLBROOK, R (1971) The inhibition and destruction of cocci. In Hugo, W R (ed) Inhibition and destruction of the microbial cell. Academic Press; London, UK; pp 369-397.

6. BOGDANOV, S (1984) Characterisation of antibacterial substances in honey. *LebensmittelWissenschaft und Technologie* 17(2): 74-76.

7. BOGDANOV, S (1989) Determination of pinocembrin in honey using HPLC. *Journal of Apicultural Research* 28(1): 55-57.

8. BOGDANOV, S; RIEDER, K; RUEGG, M (1987) Neue Qualitaskriterien bei Honiguntersuchungen. *Apidologie* 18(3): 267-278.

9. BRANIKI, F J (1981) Surgery in western Kenya. *Annals of the Royal College of Surgeons of England* 63: 348-352.

10. BREED, R S; MURRAY, E G D; HITCHENS, A P (1948) *Bergey's Manual of Determinative Bacteriology*. Williams & Wilkins; Baltimore, USA; 1529 pp (6th edition).

11. BUCHANAN, R E; GIBBONS, N E (1974) *Bergey's Manual of Determinative Bacteriology*. Williams & Wilkins; Baltimore, USA; 1246 pp (8th edition).

12. BUCHNER, R (1966) Vergleichencle Untersuchungen Ober die anti bakteriellen Wirkung von Blutenund Honigtauhonigen. *Sudwestdeutscher Imker* 18: 240-241.

13. CHAMBONNAUD, J P (1966) Etude du puvoir antibacterien des miels par une technique de diffusion en gelose. *Bulletin apicole* 9(1): 83-98.

14. CHAMBONNAUD, J P (1968) Contribution a la recherche des antibiotiques clans le miel. *Bulletin apicole* 11 (2): 133-200.

15. CHIRIFE, J; SCARMATO, G; HERSZAGE, L (1982) Scientific basis for use of granulated sugar in treatment of infected wounds. *Lancet i*: 560-561.

16. CHRISTIAN, J H B; WALTHO, I A (1964) The composition of *Staphylococcus aureus* in relation to the water activity of the growth medium. *Journal of General Microbiology* 35: 205-218.

17. CHRISTOV [KHRISTOV], G; MLADENOV, S (1961) Proprietes antimicrobiennes du miel. *Comptes rendus de la Academie bulgare des Sciences* 14(3): 303-306.

18. CHWASTEK, M (1966) Jakosc miodowpszczelich handlowych na podstavvie oznaczania ich skladnikow niecukrowcowych. czesc II. Zawartosc inhibiny w mioclach krajowych. *Rocziniki Panstwowego Zakladu Higieny* 17(1): 41-48.

19. COHEN, G; HOCHSTEIN, P (1962) Glutathione peroxidase: the major pathway for the detoxification of hydrogen peroxide in erythrocytes. American Chemical Society, 141st. Meeting, Division of Biological Chemistry. p. 58c (abstract no. 137).

20. COULTHARD, C E; MICHAELIS, R; SHORT, W F; SYKES, G; SKRIMSHIRE, G E H; STANDFAST, A F B; BIRKINSHAW, J H; RAISTRICK, H (1945) Notatin: an antibacterial glucose-aerodehydrogenase from *Penicillium notatum* Westling and *Penicillium resticulosum* sp. nov. *Biochemical Journal* 39: 2436.

21. DAGHIE, V, CIRNU, I; CIOCA, V (1971) Contribution to the study of the bacteriostatic and bactericidal action of honey produced by *Physokermes* sp. in the area of coniferous trees. Proceedings of the XXIIrd International Apicultural Congress, Moscow. Apimondia Publishing House; Bucharest, Romania; pp 593-594.

22. DAGHIE, V, CIRNU, I; CIOCA,V (1973) Contributii privind actinuea bactericida si bacteriostatica a mierii de lecaniide (*Physokermes* sp.) din zona coniferelor. *Apicultura* 26(2): 13-16.

23. DAVIS, B D; DUBELCCO, R; EISEN, H N; GINSBERG, H S; WOOD, W B (1973) *Microbiology*. Harper and Row; Hagerstown, Maryland, USA; 1562 pp (2nd edition).

24. DOLD, H; Du, D H; DZIAO, S T (1937) Nachweis antibakterieller, hitze- und lichtempfindlicher Hemmungsstoffe Inhibine im Naturhonig Blitenhonig. *Zeitschrift fur Hygiene und Infektionskrankheiten* 120: 155167.

25. DOLD, H; KNAPP, T (1949) Uber inhibierencle und modifizierencle Wirkungen des Honigs auf Diphtheriebacillen und seine Brauchbarkeit zur Bekimpfung des Diphtheriebacillentragertums. *Zeitschrift fur Hygiene und Infektionskrankheiten* 130: 323-334.

26. DOLD, H; WITZENHAUSEN, R (1955) Ein Verfahren zur Beurteilung der ortlichen inhibitorischen (keimvermehrungshemmenden) Wirkung von Honigsorten verschieclener Herkunft. *Zeitschrift fur Hygiene und Infektionskrankheiten* 141: 333-337.

27. DOLEZAL, M; DOLEZAL, M; MEORELA-KUDER, E (1988) Research on inhibine effect of herb honey. *Acta Biologica Cracoviensia Series Botanica* 30: 916.

28. DUISBERG, H; WARNECKE, B (1959) Erhitzungs-und LichteirifluB auf Fermente und Inhibine des Honigs. *Zeitschrift for Lebensmitteluntersuchurig und Forschung* 111: 111-119.

29. DRONGLERT, E (1983) A follow-up study of chronic wound healing dressing with pure natural honey. *Journal of the National Research Council of Thailand* 15(2): 39-66.

30. DUSTMANN, I H (1971) Ober die Katalaseaktivitat in Bienenhonig aus der Tracht der Heidekrautgewachse (Ericaceae). *Zeitschrift fur Lebensmitteluntersuchung undForschung* 145: 294-295.

31. DUSTMANN, J H (1972) Ober den Einfluß des Lichtes auf den PeroxidWert (Inhibin) des Honigs. *Zeitschrift fur Lebensmitteluntersuchung und Forschung* 148(5): 263-268.

32. DUSTMANN, J H (1979) Antibacterial effect honey. *Apiacta* 14(1): 711.

33. DUSTMANN, J (1987) Effect of honey on the cariogenic bacterium *Streptococcus mutans*. Proceedings of the XXXIst International Apicultural Congress of Apimondia, Warsaw, Poland. Apimondia Publishing House; Bucharest, Romania; pp 459-461.

34. FRANCO, M; Sartori, L (1940) *Sulfazione antibatterice del miele. Annali d'Igiene* 50: 216227 (abstracted in Lancet i: 1184 (1940)).

35. GAUHE, A (1941) Ober ein glukoseoxydierencles Enzym in der Pharynxdrose der Honigbiene. *Zeitschrift fur Ivergleichende Physiologie* 28(3): 211-253.

36. GONNET, M; LAVIE (1960) *Influence du chauffage Sur le facteur antibiotique present dans les miels.* Annales de l'Abeille (Paris) 3 (4): 349-364.

37. GRECEANU, A; ENCIU, V (1976) "*Observations on the antibiotic effects of propolis, pollen and honey.*" 2nd International Symposium on Apitherapy, Bucharest, Apimondia Publishing House: Bucharest, Romania; pp 177-179.

38. GROCHOWSKI, J; BILINSKA, M (1987) Biological activity of pollen, *bee bread and honey relative to selected bacterial strains.* Proceedings of the XXXIst Interriational Apicultural Congress of Apimondia, Warsaw, Poland. Apimondia Publishing House; Bucharest, Romania, pp 462.

39. GRYUNER, V S; ARINKINA, A I (1970) [Carbohydrates content, enzymatic and antimicrobial activity of honey.] *Izvestiya Vysshikh Uchebnykh Zavedenii Pishchevaya Tekhnologiya* 1970(6): 28-31 (original in Russian).

40. HAYDAK, M H; CRANE, E; DUISBERG, H; GOCHNAUER, T A; MORSE, R A; WHITE, J W, WIX, P (1975) Biological properties of honey. In Crane, E (ed) *Honey: a Comprehensive Survey.* Heinemann; London, UK; pp 258-266.

41. HODGSON, M J (1989) *Investigation of the antibacterial action spectrum of some honeys.* M Sc thesis; University of Waikato, New Zealand; 83 pp.

42. IALOMITZEANU, M; DAGHIE, V,' MIHAEScu, N F (1967) Contribution to the study of the bacteriostatic and bactericidal action of honey. Proceedings of the XXIst InternationalApicultural Congress, Budapest, Hungary. Apimondia Publishing House; Bucharest, Romania; pp 209-213.

43. IALOMITZEANU, M; DAGHIE, V (1973) Investigations of the antibiotic qualities of honey. Proceedings of the XXII/th International Apicultural Congress, Buenos Aires. Apimondia Publishing House; Bucharest, Romania; pp 438-440.

44. IBRAHIM, A S (1981) Antibacterial action of honey. Proceedings of the First International Conference on Islamic medicine. (2nd edition) (*Bulletin of Islamic Medicine,* volume 1). Kuwait Ministry of Public Health; Kuwait; pp 363-365.

45. JAMES, O B O; SEGREE, W, VENTURA, A K (1972) Some antibacterial properties of Jamaican honey. *West Indian Medical Journal* 21(7): 717.

46. JEDDAR, A; KHARSANY, A; RAMSAROOP, U G; BHAMUEE, A; HAFFEJEE, I E; MOOSA, A (1985) The antibacterial action of honey. An in vitro study. *South African Medical Journal* 67: 257-258.

47. KHRISTOV, G; MLADENOV, S (1961) Honey in surgical practice: the antibacterial properties of honey. *Khirurgiya* (Moscow) 14(10): 937-946 (original in Bulgarian).

48. LAVIE, P (1963) *Sur l'identification des substances antibacteriennes presentes dans le miel.* Comptes Rendus Academie des Sciences, Paris 256: 1858-1860.

49. LEISTNER, L; RODEL, W (1975) *The significance of water activity for microorganisms in meats.* In Duckworth, R B (ed) Water relations of foods, Academic Press; London, UK; pp 309-323.

50. LINDNER, K E (1962) Ein Beitrag zur Frage der antimikrobiellen Wirkung der Naturhonige. Zentralblatt fur Bakteriologie, *Parasitenkunde, Infektionkrankheiten und Hygiene* 115(7): 720-736.

51. LOWBURY, E J L; AYLIFFE, G A J (1974) *Drug resistance in antimicrobial therapy.* Thomas; Springfield, Illinois, USA: 211 pp.

52. MAJNO, G (1975) *The healing hand.* Man and wound in the ancient world. Harvard University Press; Cambridge, Massachusetts, USA; 571 pp.

53. MAURIZIO, A (1962) From the raw material to the finished product: honey. *Bee World* 43: 66-81.

54. MCCULLOCH, E C (1945) *Disinfection and sterilization.* Henry Kimpton; London, UK; 472 pp (2nd edition).

55. McGARRY, I P (1961) The effect of aging on the inhibitory substance in various honeys for bacteria. *Bee World* 42(2): 226-229.

56. MEIER, K E; FREITAG, G (1955) Ober die antibiotischen Eigenschaften von Sacchariden und Bienenhonig. *Zeitschrift fur Hygiene und Infektionskrankheiten* 141: 326-332.

57. MILLER, T E (1969) Killing and lysis of Gram-negative bacteria through the synergistic effect of hydrogen peroxide, ascorbic acid, and lysozyme. *Journal of Bacteriology* 98(3): 949-955.

58. MISHREF, A; MAGDA, S A; GHAZI, I M (1989) *The effect of feeding medicinal plant extracts to honeybee colonies on the antimicrobial activity of the honey produced.* Proceedings of the Fourth International Conference on Apiculture in Tropical Climates, Cairo. International Bee Research Association; London, UK; pp 80-86.

59. MIZRAHI, A; DORON, R (1982) Antimicrobial effects of hive products. *Israel Journal of Medical Sciences* 18(5): 23.

60. MOHRIG, W; MESSNER, B (1968) Lysozym als antibakteriel les Agens im Bienenhonig und Bienengift. *Acta Biologica et Medica Germanica* 21: 85-95.

61. MOLAN, P C; RUSSELL, K M (1988) Nonperoxide antibacterial activity in some New Zealand honeys. *Journal of Apicultural Research* 27(1): 62-67.

62. MOLAN, P C; SMITH, I M; REID, G M (1988) A comparison of the antibacterial activity of some New Zealand honeys. *Journal of Apicultural Research* 27(4): 252-256.

63. MOLAN, P C; ALLEN, K L; TAN, S T, WILKINS, A L (1989) *Identification of components responsible for the antibacterial activity of Manuka and Viper's Bugloss honeys* (oral paper). Annual Conference of the New Zealand Institute of Chemistry, Hamilton, New Zealand; 1989 (unpublished).

64. MORSE, R A (1986) The antibiotic properties of honey. *PanPacific Entomologist* 62(4): 370-371.

65. MOSSEL, D A A (1975) Water and microorganisms in foods a synthesis. In Duckworth, R B (ed) Water relations of foods. Academic Press; London, UK; pp 347-361.

66. NABRDALIK, M; SKARBEK, R (1974) [Inhibitory properties of bee's honey.] *Medycyna Weterynaryjna* 30(11): 669 (original in Polish).

67. NESTER, E W; ROBERTS, C E; PEARSALL, N N; MCCARTHY, B J (1978) *Microbiology.* Holt, Rinehart and Winston; New York, USA; 769 pp (2nd edition).

68. OBASEIKI-EBOR, E E; AFONYA, T C A; ONYLKWELI, A O (1983) Preliminary report on the antimicrobial activity of honey distillate. *Journal of Pharmacy and Pharmacology* 35(11): 748-749.

69. OBASEIKI-EBOR, E E; AFONYA, T C A (1984) In vitro evaluation of the anticandidiasis activity of honey distillate (HY1) compared with that of some antimycotic agents. *Journal of Pharmacy and Pharmacology* 36: 283-284.

70. PLACHY, E (1944) Studie Ober die bakterizicle Wirkung des Naturhonigs (Bluten und Blatthonig) aus verschiedenen hohenlagen sowie einige Untersuchungen Ober die Eigenschaft der antibakteriellen Hemmungstoffe (Inhibine) im Naturhonig. *Zentralblatt bir Bakteriologie* 100: 401-419.

71. POPESKOVIC, D; DAKIC, M; BUNCIC, S; Ruzic, P (1983) *A further investigation on the antimicrobial properties of honey.* Proceedings of the XXIXth International Congress of Apiculture, Budapest, Hungary. Apimondia Publishing House; Bucharest, Romania; pp 415-417.

72. POTHMANN, F J (1950) Der Einfluß von Naturhonig auf clas Wachstum der Tb.-Bakterien. *Zeitschrift fur Hygiene und Infektionskrankheiten* 130: 468484.

73. PRICA, M (1938) Ober die bactericide Wirkung des Naturhonigs. *Zeitschrift fur Hygiene und Infektionskrankheiten* 120: 437-443.

74. RADWAN, S S; EL-ESSAWY, A A; SARHAN, M M (1984) Experimental evidence for the occurrence in honey of specific substances active against microorganisms. *Zentralblatt fur Mikrobiologie* 139(4): 249-255.

75. RANSOME, H M (1937) *The Sacred Bee in Ancient Times and Folklore.* George Allen and Unwin; London, UK; 308 pp.

76. REVATHY, V, BANEFUI, S A (1980) A preliminary study of antibacterial properties of Indian honey. *Indian Journal of Biochemistry and Biophysics* 17 (supplement no. 242): 62.

77. RIZVANOV, K; BIZHEV, B (1962) [Investigation of the antibacterial

and antifungal properties of honey.] *Nauchni trudove* 11: 433443 (original in Bulgarian).

78. ROOS, D; BALM, A J M (1980) *The oxidative metabolism of monocytes.* In Sbarra, A J; Strauss, R R (ed) The reticuloendothelial system. A comprehensive treatise. Volume 2. *Biochemistry and metabolism.* Plenum Press; New York, USA; pp 189-229.

79. RUEGG, M; BLANC, B (1981) The water activity of honey and related sugar solutions. *LebensmittelWissenschaft und Technologie* 14: 16.

80. RUSSELL, K M (1983) *The antibacterial properties of honey.* M Sc thesis University of Waikato; New Zealand; 147 pp.

81. RUSSELL, K M; MOLAN, P C; WILKINS, A L; HOLLAND, P T (1988) Identification of some antibacterial constituents of New Zealand manuka honey. *Journal of Agricultural and Food Chemistry* 38: 10-13.

82. RYCHLIK, M; DOLEZAL, M (1961) Wlasciwosci inhibinowe niekterych miod6w Polskich6. *Pszczelnicze Zeszyty Naukowe* 5(2): 53-64.

83. SACKETT; W G (1919) Honey as a carrier of intestinal diseases. *Bulletin of the Colorado State University Agricultural Experimental Station* No. 252: 18 pp.

84. SCHADE, J E; MARSH, G L; ECKERT, J E (1958) Diastase activity and hydroxymethylfurfural in honey and their usefulness in detecting heat alteration. *Food Research* 23: 446-463.

85. SCHEPARTZ, A I (1966) Honey catalase: occurrence and some kinetic properties. *Journal of Apicultural Research* 5(3): 167-176.

86. SCHEPARTZ, A I (1966) The glucoseoxidase of honey. IV. Some additional observations. *Biochimica et Biophysica Acta* 118: 637-640.

87. SCHEPARTZ, A I; SUBERS, M H (1964) The glucoseoxidase of honey. 1. Purification and some general properties of the enzyme. *Siochimica et Biophysica Acta* 85: 228-237.

88. SCHEPARTZ, A I; SUBERS, M H (1966) Catalase in honey. *Journal of Apicultural Research* 5(l): 37-43.

89. SCHULER, R; VOGEL, R (1956) Wirkstoffe des Bienenhonigs. *Arzneimittel Forschung* 6: 661-663.

90. SCOTT, W J (1957) Water relations of food spoilage microorganisms. *Advances in Food Research* 7: 83-127.

91. SEDOVA, N N; USMANOV, M F (1973) [Antimicrobial properties of some types of honey from Uzbekistan.] *Vdprosy Pitaniya* 32(2): 84-85 (original in Russian).

92. SHANSON, D C (1989) *Microbiology in Clinical Practice.* Wright; London, UK; 657 pp (2nd edition).

SKRYPNIK, E I; KHOROCSKII, L N (1974) [Persistence of tuberculosis in honeys]. *Pchelovadstvo* 94(5): 41 (original in Russian).

93. SMITH, M R; MCCAUGHEY, W F; KEMMERER, A R (1969) Biological effects of honey. *Journal of Apicultural Research* 8(2): 99-110.

94. STINSON, E E; SUBERS, M H; PETTY, J; WHITE, J W (1960) The composition of honey. V. Separation and identification of the organic acids. *Archives of Biochemistry and Biophysics* 89: 612.

95. STOMFAYSTITZ, J; KOMINOS, S D (1960) Ober bakteriostatische Wirkung des honigs. *Zeitschrift fur Lebensmitteluntersuchung und Forschung* 113: 304-309.

96. SYKES, G (1965) *Disinfection and Sterilization.* Spon; London, UK; 486 pp (2nd edition).

97. TAN, S T (1989) *A chemical investigation of some New Zealand honeys.* D Phil thesis; University of Waikato; New Zealand; 201 pp.

98. THIMANN, K V (1963) *The Life of Bacteria.* Macmillan; New York; 909 pp (2nd edition).

99. TOMLINSON, J T, WILLIAMS, S C (1985) Antibiotic properties of honey produced by the domestic honey bee *Apis mellifera* (Hymenoptera: Apiclae). *PanPacific Entomologist* 610): 346-347.

100. TOTH, G; LEMBERKOVICS, E; KUTASISZABO, J (1987) The volatile components of some Hungarian honeys and their antimicrobial effects. *American Bee Journal* 127(7): 496-497.

101. TYSSET, C; DURAND, C (1973) De la survie de quelques germes Gram negatif, non sporules, dans le miels du commerce. *Bulletin de l'Academie Veterinaire de France* 46(4): 191-196.

102. TYSSET, C; DURAND, C (1976) De la survie de quelques enter-obacteries dans le miel stocke dans une enceinte refrigere a +10= C. *Bulletin de l'Academie Veterinaire de France* 49(4): 417-422.

103. TYSSET, C; ROUSSEAU, M; DURAND, C (1980) Microbism and wholesomeness of commercial honey. *Apiacta* 15(2): 51-60.

104. VERGT, I (1951) Lactivite antibacterienne de la propolis du miel et de la gelee royale. *Apiculteur* 95(6: Section scientificque): 13-20.

105. WAITES, W M; BAYLISS, C E; KING, N R; DAVIES, A M C (1979) The effect of transitional metal ions on the resistance of bacterial spores to hydrogen peroxide and to heat. *Journal of General Microbiology* 112: 225-233.

106. WARNECKE, B; DUISBERG, H (1958) Die bakteriostatische (inhibitorische) *Wirkungs des Honigs, Zeitschrift fur Lebensmitteluntersuchung und ForSchung* 107: 340.

107. WARNECKE, B; DUISBERG, H (1964) Die Erhaltung der Honiginhibine durch Ausschaltung des UVLichtes. *Zeitschrift fur Lebensmitteluntersuchung und Forschung* 124: 265-270.

108. WELLFORD, T E T; EADIE, T, LLEWELLYN, G C (1978) Evaluating the inhibitory action of honey on fungal growth, sporulation and aflatoxin pro-duction. *Zeitschrift for Lebensmitteluntersuchung und Forschung* 166(5): 280-283.

109. WHITE, J W; SUBERS, M H; SCHEPARTZ, A I (1962) The identifi-cation of inhibine. *American Bee Journal* 102(11): 430-431.

110. WHITE, J W; SUBERS, M H; SCHEPARTZ, A I (1963) The identification of Inhibine, the antibacterial factor in honey, as hydrogen peroxide and its origin in a honey glucoseoxidase system. *Biochimica et Biophysica Acta* 73: 57-70.

111. WHITE, J W; SUBERS, M H (1963) Studies on honey Inhibine. 2. A chemical assay. *Journal of Apicultural Research* 2(2): 93-100.

112. WHITE, J W; SUBERS, M H (1964) Studies on honey Inhibine. 3. Effect of heat. *Journal of Apicultural Research* 3(1): 45-50.

113. WHITE, I W; SUBERS, M H (1964) Studies on honey Inhibine. 4. Destruction of the peroxide accumulation system by light. *Journal of Food Science* 29(6): 819-828.

114. WILLIX, D J (1991) *A comparative study of the antibacterial action spectrum of manuka honey and other honey.* M Sc thesis; University of Waikato; New Zealand; 112 pp.

115. WOOTON, M; EDWARDS, R A; ROWSE, A (1978) Antibacterial properties of some Australian honeys. *Food Technology in Australia* (May): 175-176.

116. YATSUNAMI, K; ECHIGO, T (1984) [Antibacterial action of honey and royal jelly.] *Honeybee Science* 5(3): 125-130. (original in Japanese).

117. YOIRISH, N (1977) *Curative Properties of Honey & Bee Venom.* New Glide Publications: San Francisco, USA; 198 pp.

118. ZOMLA, A; LULAT, A (1989) Honey a remedy rediscovered. *Journal of the Royal Society of Medicine* 82: 384-385.

The following references are from Molan, P. "Potential of Honey in the Treatment of Wounds and Burns." *Am. J. Clin. Dermatology* 2, no. 1 (2001): 13-19.

Blomfield, E. "Old Remedies." *J.R. Coll. Gen. Pract.* 26 (1976): 576.

Dunford, C., R.A. Cooper, P.C. Molan. "Using Honey as a Dressing for Infected Skin Wounds." *Nurs. Times* 96 (NT PLUS) (2000): 7-9.

Kaufman, T., R.A. Neuman, A. Weinberg. "Is Postburn Dermal Ischaemia Enhanced by Oxygen-free Radicals?" *Burns* 15, no. 5 (1989): 291-294.

McInerney, R.J.F. "Honey—a Remedy Rediscovered." *J. R. Soc. Med.* 83 (1990): 127.

Other Sources and Web Sites

Other source books used include the following:

Honey and Healing (2001) International Bee Research Assn. (IBRA) 18 North Road, Cardiff, CF10 3DT, United Kingdom ($10). 50 pages.

This book incorporates Molan's two most recent *Bee World* reviews along with six other chapters by different authors. If you only get one other book on honey as a medicine, this is the one you should get.

Eva Crane's trilogy:
Honey, A Comprehensive Survey (1979) London: Heinemann.
The World History of Beekeeping and Honey Hunting (1999) New York: Routledge.
The Archaeology of Beekeeping (1983) London: Duckworth.

Dr. Crane, first director of the International Bee Research Assn., built a strong foundation with these books that many have used. They are considered the bibles of honey.

Two U.S. books provide a world of information on honey and bees (they are revised every so often, so get the latest edition):
Joe Graham, ed. *The Hive and the Honey Bee* (1992 ed.) Hamilton, IL: Dadant & Sons.
Root, A.I. et al. *ABC and XYZ of Bee Culture* (1972 ed.) Medina, OH: A.I. Root Co.

Three books that provide good anecdotal tales on the medicinal benefits of honey (with an occasional dollop of science) are:
Honey and Health (1938) by Bodog Beck. New York: Robert McBride Co.
Folk Medicine (1958) by Dr. D.C. Jarvis. New York: Fawcett Crest Books (Holt, Rinehart and Winston).
Bees Don't Get Arthritis (1979) by Fred Malone. New York: Dutton.

One other reference book is a combination of anecdotes and science:
Curative Properties of Honey and Bee Venom (1977) by N. Yoirish. San Francisco: New Glide Publications. (translated from a Russian version that appeared in Moscow in 1959)

Yoirish describes a number of apparently reputable Soviet studies on the medicinal benefits of honey. I have included some herein, but have reluctantly chosen to put them under the heading of anecdotes because Soviet science in the first half of the 20th Century is suspect due to a few documented cases of fraudulent data. It is unforntuate that the misdeeds of a few should cast a cloud of suspicion over all Soviet science (that the Russians were first in space speaks volumes for their science), but that is the way things are. I'm probably being unfair to the Soviet scientist mentioned by Yoirish, as well (Alas, poor Yoirish, I know you well).

For those readers with an interest in commercial beekeeping in the U.S., the May 1993 *National Geographic* tells a good story in pictures and words. Commercial beekeepers spend a lot of time on the road as they truck their bees from one flower source to another. City-dwellers with only one or two hives enjoy the luxury of keeping their bees at one site year-round.

Following are ten references from the 1990s, not included in Molan's reviews. These are from an IBRA publication of abstracts, IBRA Bibliography, *Honey in Medicine*, 1990-1995. Cardiff, U.K.: IBRA, 1996.

Armstrong, S., G.W. Otis. "The Antibacterial Properties of Honey." *Bee Culture* 123, no. 9 (1995): 500-502.

Boenarchuk, L.E. et al. "The Effects of Honey, Pollen and Some Plant Products on the Health of People in Areas of Chronic Radioactive Pollution." *Bdzhil'nitstvo* 21 (1994): 66-69.

Croft, L.R. Honey and Hay Fever: *A Report on the Treatment of Hay Fever with Honey*. Salford, U.K.; L.R. Croft. 35 pp.

Kaigi, C. "Heilmittel Honig [Honey for Healing]." *Schweizerische Bienen-Zeitung* 118, no. 10 (1995): 590-592. At this hospital in Solothurn, Switzerland, honey has been successfully used in the treatment of leg ulcers, decubitus sores (pressure wounds) furuncles, abscesses, fistulas, etc. Some examples, including treatment of chronic wounds are described, with photographs.

Pereira, P.C. et al. "Use of Honey as Nutritional and Therapeautic Supplement in the Treatment of Infectious Diseases." *Journal of Venomous Animals and Toxins* 1, no. 2 (1995): 87-88.

Postmes, T. Honey Dressings for Burns; A Two-way Approach. Maastricht, Netherlands; (Ed. 2); 81 pp.

Quddus, A.S.M.R. "Natural Honey Prevents Indomethiacin- and Ethanol-induced Lesions in Rats." *Saudi Medical Journal* 13, no. 5 (1992): 464.

Rieder, K. "Wundbehandlung mit Honig [Wound Treatment with Honey]." *Schweizerishce Bienen-Zeitung* 118, no. 10 (1995): 579.

Sala-Llinares, A. "Apicultura y fitoerapia. Utilizacion de los productos apicolas en diversas formulas fitoterapeuticas [Beekeeping and phytotherapy: use of bee-keeping products in various phytotherapeutic formations]." *Vida Apicola* No. 70 (1995): 12-16.

Willix, D.J. *The Marketing of Honey as a Medicine. A Report for the Beekeeper's Association of New Zealand.* (1991): iii + 48 pp.

Listed below are a number of very good web sites:

International Bee Research Association (IBRA)
www.ibra.org.uk
IBRA holds the world's largest storehouse of information on bees and honey. Their web site has links to other informative sites.

Peter Molan, University of Waikato
http://honey.bio.waikato.ac.nz
Excellent site for the latest on the medicinal benefits of honey.

National Honey Board
www.nhb.org
www.honey.com
The latest information on all aspects of honey. Good links to other sites.

Miscellaneous
www.beesource.com/pov/traynor/index.htm
Dr. Barry Birkey, W. Chicago, Illinois, has set up POV (point of view) websites for myself and several other bee people. A mix of information is included on these sites.

Index

RM   Traynor, Joe.
666
.H55   Honey
T73
2002

	DATE DUE		

HO
The
Me

TO OR

BookN
30

www
www

ASK

Lake Tahoe Community College
Library & Media Services
So. Lake Tahoe, CA 96150